The Terrain Is Everything

by

Susan Stockton

copyright 2000

The Terrain Is Everything
by
Susan Stockton

Copyright 2000 by Susan Stockton

All Rights Reserved
Printed in the United States of America
2nd Printing - 2002

ISBN 0-9628770-1-8

Library of Congress Catalog Number: 00-192255

The Terrain is Everything is not intended as medical advice. It is written solely for informational and educational purposes. Please consult a health professional should the need for one be indicated.

Power of One Publishing
c/o Renew Life
2076 Sunnydale Blvd.
Clearwater, FL 33765-1201
1-800-830-4778, ext. 246

DEDICATION

This book is dedicated to my beloved late son,
Michael David Swimmer

ACKNOWLEDGMENTS

I am hugely indebted to my dear friend, Jack Spence, AP, for making this book possible. The time he spent scanning text, loading programs and patiently helping me to become computer literate is most appreciated. Without his help and encouragement, and the loving support of his wife "Well," this book would never have become a reality. *And,* were it not for Sandy Knowles, her plethora of skills and ideas — and her big heart — I'd not have been able to transform the manuscript into a book. These are the angels in my life who have helped not only move my work forward but turn my life around. I am profoundly grateful!

I must acknowledge, too, those who contributed so heavily to the production of my first book, a forerunner to this one. A big "thank you" to Penny Jensen, wherever you are now, a decade later, for your fine illustrations which were so generously contributed. A very special acknowledgment goes to a very special friend, the late Bryant Gardner, my dear companion and helper, who was always there to listen, to assist, to support and inspire.

I am indebted, as well, to Ruth Swimmer and Judy Koster, RN, for patiently proofreading this and other manuscripts.

Finally, I want to thank Kenn and Viola Rust for their fine work in preparing the manuscript for the second printing.

TABLE OF CONTENTS

INTRODUCTION

My first book, *The Book of Health,* was published in 1990 as an outgrowth of my teaching activity. It was basically a compilation of lecture notes from my *Health Care Alternatives* classes which I'd begun teaching in 1988. In 1997, I revised it somewhat, adding postscripts to the end of chapters as a means of updating and amending the text. I was never happy with this format (nor all of the content), however, and have long wanted to redo the entire book. Late in 1999, on the heels of a series of publishing disasters involving *The Book of Health* and others, the way was cleared for me to not only rewrite that book, but to integrate into it selected information and excerpts from many of my other writings.

The Terrain is Everything therefore has emerged as an updated synthesis of some of the most important information I've gathered since beginning my natural healing studies many years ago. In it you'll find information from *The Natural Healing Perspective; Acupuncture: The Manipulation of Subtle Energies, the Restoration of Health* and *The Book of Health.* The information in these books is tied together with a common theme: The **terrain**, which encompasses the internal environment of the physical body, the external expression of it in structural form and the subtle energy composition holding it all together, will dictate our level of well-being. Pathological alterations in this terrain will lead to imbalances — energetic, structural, biochemical and microbial imbalances — which, in turn, will create disease conditions. The most effective treatments, therefore, are those that initiate favorable changes in the terrain, restoring dynamic balance on all levels of being.

The Terrain is Everything defines the natural healing perspective, comparing and contrasting it with the medical model. It also identifies and explores major "contextual" factors (those making up the context, or environment, in which we exist) that can move us in the direction of disease. The natural healing perspective views disease causation as multifactorial, while the medical model, through application of the "scientific method," studies single variables as suspected causes of disease. The factors influencing our health are numerous. Some are obvious; some are subtle.

All stem from the "context" in which we live our lives and which dictates the condition of the terrain of our bodies. Therefore, all factors must be considered. A 'holistic' approach to healing, one that takes into account the many variables which influence our health, and the many modalities which can be used to maintain and restore it, is vitally important. It is a limited, myopic and erroneous oversimplification to view microbes as the cause of disease, for reasons explored within this book. As we enter the new millennium, a paradigm shift is occurring, as more and more of us awaken to Louis Pasteur's deathbed realization, "The microbe is nothing. **The terrain is everything.**"

CHAPTER 1

The Natural Healing Perspective

"Holism is essentially contextualism."
Walene James

We in the United States are spending a tremendous amount of money annually on health care, close to two trillion dollars per year. Between 1980 and 1990, health care costs rose 117%, and the cost of drugs rose a staggering 152%, while general inflation was only 58%.(1) Most of the money being spent on health care today in this country is being spent on allopathic medicine. Allopathic medicine is chemically-based medicine, the cornerstone of Western medical practice which features drugs and surgery as its major modalities.

Americans are avid consumers of drugs. We pop over 25 million pills *per hour.* And, three out of four of the pills we consume routinely are immunosuppressive in their effect, which is to say that they actually *suppress* our immune systems, reduce our resistance.

One would think, in view of our liberal expenditures on health care, that we must be a very healthy nation. Not so. At one time we were. In 1900, America was the healthiest nation in the world. By 1920, we had dropped down to second place, and by 1978, according to statistics compiled by the National Bureau of Health Statistics, we had dropped down to 79th place (out of 93 industrialized nations).(2) Dropping at this rate, it is plain to see that by now we are at or near the very bottom. America is now on a par with third world nations when it comes to our health despite our great wealth. The situation today is that every third person is allergic to something; every fifth person is mentally ill; every thirty seconds someone dies of a heart attack, and every fifty-five seconds someone dies of cancer.

Cancer has become the number one childhood killer, barring accidents(3) ... the *number one childhood killer!* The "war on cancer" began many years ago, during the Nixon administration. It's a war we are clearly losing, for the incidence of cancer in the United States increased by 48% between 1950 and 1990. We are not losing this war due to lack of funds, however, for the National Cancer Institute spends over $3 million dollars *every single day* on research. Cancer is big business in this country. It's been said there are more people making a living on cancer than there are dying from it. The money spent on cancer research goes largely into *drug* research because the funding for it is provided by ... guess who? The drug companies!

In 1991, a German biostatistician, Ulrich Abel, did a survey of oncologists (cancer doctors). He asked them what they would do if they or a loved one developed cancer. Interestingly, over 50% of them said they would *not* submit to chemotherapy nor would they advise their loved ones to do so. These are the same doctors who are *ordering chemotherapy for their patients*. And they are saying they would not use it on themselves or their families! Doesn't that tell us something?

Another interesting study was done by a veteran cancer researcher, Dr. Hardin Jones. Dr. Jones, affiliated with the University of California, decided at one point to do a study no one else had ever done. He did follow-up on patients who did not listen to the advice of their doctors. These were cancer patients who were told they needed to have chemotherapy, surgery or radiation, and rather than do that, they just ignored the diagnosis of cancer. They didn't go for alternative therapies; they just did nothing. Dr. Jones compared this group of people to another group diagnosed with cancer who were compliant with their treatment recommendations, who *did* have the chemo, the surgery, the radiation. Which group do you suppose lived longer? It was the group that did nothing! That group not only lived longer, but the shocking thing is they lived up to *four times* longer than those who submitted to standard therapy. I cite this study, not to recommend that the cancer patient refuse all treatment, but to suggest s/he choose wisely and know the available alternatives.

Medicine is failing to cure not only cancer but also a number of other diseases. Bear in mind, however, that medicine is not really in the business of *curing* disease, not if we construe the word "cure" to mean identification and correction of the basic cause of the disease. What medicine *is* in the business of doing is alleviating symptoms. There is certainly nothing wrong with alleviating symptoms. We all seek relief from pain when it overwhelms us. However, utilizing the tools of drugs and surgery to alleviate symptoms often means the alleviation is accomplished by means of suppression. And, by suppressing symptoms rather than correcting their cause, we tend to set ourselves up for the development of more serious problems later. Such thinking is the basis of homotoxicology.

Homotoxicology is the study of how disease progresses in the body. This progression frequently begins, ironically, at the point at which many consider themselves to be "cured" of an ailment, for the cure, all too often, is nothing more than a suppression of disagreeable symptoms. Such symptoms are, in fact, the expression of the body's own healing mechanism at work. It is a basic tenet of homotoxicology that the body's reactions of symptom formation are goal-oriented and precipitate the reversal of the disease process — i.e., acute conditions such as inflammation, skin eruptions or diarrhea are signs not of sickness but of healing-in-process. This self-healing process is essentially a self-cleansing process, for it is the presence of 'homotoxins' (toxic substances against which the body defends itself) in the system that is the basic cause of disease.

The use of allopathic medicine may result in the suppression of annoying acute symptoms, but in the long run it can also set the stage for development of chronic degenerative disease, for drugs are toxins. When they are used to destroy bacteria, the bacterial corpses (or endotoxins) unite with the body's own proteins, as well as with molecules of the drug itself, and form what are called "wild peptides" or "false proteins." The body identifies these as 'non-self' molecules and produces substances to combat them. The natural consequence is the development of an allergic reaction and/or autoimmune disease.

The father of homotoxicology, Hans Heinrich Reckeweg, a homeopathic (natural medicine) medical doctor, was born in Germany in 1905. The recovery of his father from a serious degenerative disease through homeopathy in 1923 prompted Reckeweg to seek to unite his studies of medicine and homeopathy. In 1955, he wrote his first book on homotoxins.

Reckeweg developed a comprehensive table of "homotoxicosis" which defines and details the progression of disease. The first three **"humoral"** phases of the disease process consist of **excretion, reaction** and **deposition.** It is in these phases that the detoxification and elimination of homotoxins occur. The last three **"cellular"** phases encompass constitutional diseases of a lingering nature and consist of **impregnation, degeneration** and **neoplasm** (cancer) phases. These sets of three phases each are divided by an imaginary line called a "biological section," as illustrated in the table of homotoxicosis, chart 1A.

The prognosis of any disease within the first three phases is decidedly favorable, while those in cellular phases hold a more guarded prognosis. In the humoral phases, the body's enzymes remain intact, and self-healing activity is in progress, while beyond the biological section, in the cellular phases, enzymes have become impaired. The trend is therefore toward deterioration. Even at this stage, however, reversal of the disease is possible, provided allopathic drugs are not administered.

A disorder in the humoral phase, such as tonsillitis (a reaction phase disorder), can progress into a variety of illnesses with completely different symptoms such as epilepsy, asthma, nephrosis, diabetes or even sarcoma. Development in this manner, from the left to the right side of the chart, is known as **progressive vicariation.** Regression can also occur — i.e., movement from right to left, or from cellular phase to humoral phase. This is true healing, but unfortunately is most often not recognized as such, being viewed rather as the development of another illness. Movement in this backwards direction is known as **regressive vicariation.** An example of regressive vicariation would be the movement of a viral infection (impregnation phase) into a fever (reaction phase). A fever is always a favorable sign, for, according to Nobel prize winner Professor Lwoff of Paris, viruses are killed by the temperature increase. As body temperature increases, metabolism also increases, with white blood cells traveling through the body at a greatly accelerated speed, killing germs as they go.

According to Reckeweg, biological therapy (homeopathy) promotes regressive vicariation, while retoxic therapy (allopathic medicine) promotes progressive vicariation. Stated in another way, homeopathy induces "healing crisis" through the retracing of disease symptoms; allopathic medicine extinguishes the *appearance* of disease, while simultaneously creating new homotoxins that give rise to pathological processes and move us into cellular phases of the disease process (away from healing, rather than toward it).

IATROGENIC DISEASE

Ironically, in its very effort to alleviate symptoms by suppressing them, the medical profession has produced an entirely new category of disease known as *iatrogenic* disease. The word "iatrogenic" means physician-induced. This is not to say that doctors are going around intentionally making people sick. Iatrogenic disorders are those that result from allopathic treatment, side effects from drugs and surgery.

"The Wisdom of Allopathic Medicine," a true story originally published in the January 1974 edition of a magazine called *Share* appears on page 6. It deals with the topic of iatrogenic disorder.

A young man developed a sore throat. He went to his physician who prescribed penicillin for the inflammation. The sore throat promptly disappeared. Three days later, however, he developed itching and hives all over his body. The physician correctly diagnosed a penicillin reaction and prescribed an antihistamine. The hives went away. The antihistamine caused the patient to be drowsy so that he cut his hand while at work. He went to the company's nurse who put some antibacterial salve on it. The salve contained penicillin and caused the hives to return. Recognizing a possible serious anaphylactic reaction for the second time, his physician then prescribed corticosteroids (cortisone). The hives again disappeared.

Unfortunately, the patient developed abdominal pains and noted blood in his stool. The correct diagnosis was then made of a bleeding peptic ulcer brought on by the cortisone. The patient failed to respond to standard measures to correct the hemorrhage, so the next course of action indicated was a partial gastrectomy. The surgery was successful. The stomach pains diminished, and the bleeding stopped. The patient lost so much blood due to the hemorrhaging in the stomach that a transfusion was indicated. He was administered two pints of blood and promptly contracted hepatitis as a result of the transfusion.

But, being young and vital, he recovered from the hepatitis. However, at the point of insertion of the transfusion needle, a painful red swelling appeared, indicating a probable infection. Having had a previous bad experience with penicillin, the drug of choice for this infection became tetracycline. The infection promptly subsided.

The disruption of the intestinal bacteria by the tetracycline caused painful abdominal spasms and severe diarrhea. The patient was then administered an antispasmodic type of drug, and the diarrhea and spasms then subsided. Unfortunately, the drug was in the belladonna, or muscle relaxing group of drugs, which relaxed the smooth muscles all over the body. From this action on the iris of the eye, it impaired the patient's vision. He drove his car into a tree and was instantly killed.

This true story is an extreme one, to be sure. This young man initially had a sore throat; one thing led to another, and he ended up dead. Although extreme and unusual, this story does serve to underscore a point. The point is that when we suppress a symptom here, another is going to pop up there, and when we suppress it there, another one is going to pop up somewhere else, and so on and so on.

Iatrogenic disorders are a growing problem today. "Statistics show that once you check into a hospital, you have a 1 in 15 chance of experiencing an adverse drug reaction and, even worse, a 1 in 312 chance that the reaction will prove fatal.[4] About the same number of people now die from reactions to prescription medications as from car accidents.(5) In 1988, the Government Accounting Office did a study which showed that prescription drugs killed as many as 140,000 people that year: That's 384 people dying every day of the side effects of prescription medications — seven times more people than die from the use of street drugs. A Harvard medical study done in 1996 listed conventional medical care as the fourth leading cause of death in this country.(6)

I think the most telling statistics I have encountered anywhere have had to do with doctors' strikes. It seems that every time and everywhere that medical doctors go on strike, refusing to treat anything but traumatic cases, the mortality rate (the death rate) drops, sometimes dramatically; most dramatically was in Israel in 1973 when the doctors went on strike for two months. During that period of time, the death rate **fell 50%.** They say morticians were complaining that business had not been that bad in twenty years — since the *last* doctors' strike!

To end this section, another statistical gem: Only 10-20% of all procedures currently in use in medical practice have been shown by controlled trial to be efficacious.(7) This is a rather shocking finding in a profession that prides itself on being "scientific."

SIGNS OF CHANGE

Despite its shortcomings, the medical monopoly has enjoyed a long-time reign in this country and in most of the world, but I am happy to report that the tides are turning. They began noticeably turning in August, 1987, when the American Medical Association was found guilty of conspiring to destroy the chiropractic profession. The AMA appealed the decision, and in February 1990, they lost their appeal case. As a consequence of their action, the AMA was told they would have to publicly apologize to the chiropractors. And so, in the January 13, 1992 edition of the JAMA (*Journal of the American Medical Association*), the full text of the judge's injunction order against the AMA was published. That hardly constituted a public apology, since most of us do not read the JAMA, and, indeed, don't even know the trial took place! Now, you would think that to be big news, wouldn't you?: the AMA found guilty of conspiring to destroy their competition. But, for some reason, it just didn't get a lot of press...

Another encouraging sign of change is that in 1992, the year that the AMA apologized to the chiropractors, the Office of Alternative Medicine was established as a branch of the National Institute of Health. It was set up to do research on alternative treatment modalities. Their initial budget was a mere $2 million dollars, just a drop in the bucket compared to the overall budget of the National Institute of Health, which was about $10 billion dollars. However, three years later, in 1995, the Office of Alternative Medicine had been given a $13 million dollar budget. More funds are continually being allocated for the study of alternative treatment. Another encouraging change is that, as of 1995, six states had enacted medical freedom laws: Alaska, Washington, North Carolina, Oklahoma, Oregon and New York. These states have passed legislation to protect the alternative disciplines.

Yet another sign that the tides are turning is the fact that there are now three accredited naturopathic colleges in this country and eleven states that license naturopaths: New Hampshire, Montana, Alaska, Arizona, Connecticut, Hawaii, Oregon, Utah, Washington, Vermont and Maine. We can be encouraged by the fact that, as of 1996, thirty-four American medical schools (of 125), including Yale and Harvard, were offering courses in what they call "complementary medicine." Complementary medicine is another word for alternative medicine. (Medicine used to call it "alternative," but when it began to become popular, it was designated as "complementary" instead.)

Perhaps the most encouraging sign of change is the fact that the majority of us, we the people, say we are dissatisfied with medicine as it is practiced today, and we see a need for change. According to a landmark study done in 1993 by the Harvard Medical School and published in the *New England Journal of Medicine*, one out of every three Americans were, at that time, seeking alternative health care, and we were making 10% more office visits annually to alternative practitioners than to the medical ones. By 1998 more Americans had visited alternative doctors than medical ones.[8]

THE DISEASE MODEL: TWO PERSPECTIVES

To understand natural healing principles, it is useful to contrast them with those of the medical model or allopathic paradigm. When we talk about the medical model, we are talking basically about the germ theory. We are all familiar with the germ theory. It simply states that specific diseases are caused by specific germs.

The roots of the germ theory go back to the middle of the 19th century to the country of France, to that well-known scientist, Louis Pasteur. Pasteur taught us that germs are airborne and that specific germs cause specific diseases. The germ theory is based on the notion that germs are *monomorphic*. Monomorphic means "one form." The monomorphic doctrine states that germs are fixed in form, that they do not change their form or identity over the course of a lifetime. In other words, a germ of a particular sort, let's say an E. coli bacillus, is today an E. coli bacillus, was yesterday an E. coli bacillus and will be one tomorrow as well. The germ does not have the ability to change into anything else, according to the monomorphic doctrine. A corollary to the germ theory is that if we find the right drug to destroy the germ or microorganism associated with the specific disease, then we will successfully cure that disease.

The natural healing model asserts that the basic cause of disease is autointoxication. Autointoxication is a state where the body is overwhelmed by the toxins retained by it as a result of faulty diet, poor digestion, poor elimination and poor liver function. The concept of autointoxication is well articulated in the words of Stanley Burroughs in his classic, *Healing for the Age of Enlightenment:*

> Disease, old age and death are the result of accumulated poisons and congestion throughout the body. These toxins become crystallized and hardened, settling around the joints, in the muscles and throughout the billions of cells all over the body.
>
> It is presumed by orthodox medicine that we have perfectly healthy bodies until something, such as germs and viruses, comes along to destroy it, whereas actually the building materials for organs and cells are defective, and thus they are inferior or diseased.
>
> Germs, in fact, are our friends, and, if given a chance, will break up and consume these large amounts of waste matter and assist us in eliminating them from the body. These germs and viruses exist in excess only when we provide a breeding ground in which they can multiply.
>
> Germs and viruses are in the body to help break down waste material and can do no harm to healthy tissue.
>
> One of nature's most effective methods of cleansing the body is to start loosening and eliminating these poisons with bacterial action. As this action progresses, we become sick and feverish; large amounts

of mucous are eliminated; diarrhea increases the discharge of waste material; and all of our resources go into action to clean out as fast as possible to prevent these poisons from killing us. **INFECTIONS ARE NOT CAUGHT — THEY ARE CREATED BY NATURE TO ASSIST IN BURNING OUR SURPLUS WASTE.**

Here we find expression of Reckeweg's notion that symptom formation in the body is goal-oriented, and that goal is healing through cleansing. The acute symptoms we so often seek to suppress can be rightly viewed therefore, not as illness, but as a temporary "cleansing reaction" or "healing crisis" and should be welcomed as a sign of healing-in-progress and not suppressed. We should not try to cure a cure! Germs, Burroughs tells us, do not initiate a diseased state but appear *after* the person has become ill.

The natural healing model does not deny the existence of germs — that would be rather like asserting that the world is flat — but, it does maintain that germs are (as Burroughs said) basically our friends and do no harm in the healthy body. They do, in fact, serve constructive purpose, causing no harm until, and unless, conditions within the body shift, causing the germs to multiply — not only to multiply but to change form.

The idea that germs actually have the ability to change form is part and parcel of the **pleomorphic doctrine.** The pleomorphic doctrine is exactly the opposite of the monomorphic doctrine. The monomorphic doctrine says germs are fixed in form, and the pleomorphic doctrine says germs are form-changing. According to the pleomorphic doctrine, what is an E. coli bacillus today, might yesterday have been a bacteria of a different strain and might begin tomorrow to shift into an entirely different microorganism, into a viral or a fungal form perhaps, according to changes in the *terrain* or internal environment of the host organism.

The roots of the pleomorphic doctrine take us back in time once again to the country of France and once again to the middle of the 1800s — this time to the work of a contemporary of Louis Pasteur, Antoine Béchamp. Béchamp is not well-known. He is not well-known because his findings challenge the very foundation of modern medicine and therefore have been suppressed.

We know of the work of Antoine Béchamp largely through the efforts of a woman named Ethyl Douglas Hume who wrote a book entitled *Béchamp or Pasteur? A Lost Chapter in the History of Biology* at the end of the 19th century. This book was published in the early 1900s in England and had long been out of print until relatively recently when it surfaced under another title. It's based on information which Hume took from the personal memoirs of both French scientists and from the notes of the scientific academies of the day.

According to Hume's research, Antoine Béchamp was a learned man of science who was well-respected by his peers. He had impressive scientific credentials; was a Doctor of Science, a Doctor of Medicine, a master pharmacologist and professor who taught classes in chemistry, toxicology, physics and pharmacy. Béchamp did not seek notoriety but rather sought to unravel the mysteries of life. And, toward that end, spent hour after hour at work in his laboratory with his microscope.

Pasteur, on the other hand, according to Hume's findings, was a chemist and, if the truth be known, a second-rate scientist who was not well-respected by his peers. He was, however, very popular with the people, for he was quite close to the reigning monarchy of the time, Napoleon. Pasteur had a flair for self-promotion and a love of the limelight, and he sought to further his career at all costs, according to Hume.

One of the most shocking things we learn about Pasteur from Hume's research is that some of the most important scientific discoveries with which history credits him were, in fact, discoveries which were made by his brilliant contemporary, Antoine Béchamp. Pasteur was essentially a plagiarist, claiming as his own many of the findings of Béchamp. Ironically, the very germ theory which was developed by Pasteur was an outgrowth of his misinterpretation of some of the early experiments of Antoine Béchamp. Hume gives details in her book.

While Béchamp's experiments built a convincing case for the validity of pleomorphism, he did not have available to him in his time the technology that would allow him to actually witness pleomorphic activity. He could not look into his microscope and actually see microorganisms changing into other microorganisms. The technology which would allow one to witness pleomorphic activity would not come onto the scene until about twenty years after the death of Antoine Béchamp. That technology was introduced in the late 1920s in the United States by another brilliant man whose work has been largely suppressed. That man was Royal Raymond Rife.

PROOF OF PLEOMORPHISM

Rife was not a doctor. He was an inventor. He invented an incredible light-source microscope capable of super-magnification which allowed the viewer to actually witness the activity of living microorganisms with complete clarity. This is something that not even the most powerful conventional microscopes of today can do. We have electron microscopes that are very powerful in terms of providing super-magnification; however, one cannot view living microorganisms underneath these microscopes. The microorganism must be dead. It must be dead in order to be stained so that it may be made visible. The technology that Rife used to build his microscope was light years ahead of his time. Using his remarkable microscope, Rife found that when he changed the medium or the environment (the *terrain)* in which the microorganisms lived, he actually changed the identity of the microorganisms. In other words, he verified pleomorphic activity with the aid of his microscope. Rife was not the only person to witness pleomorphic activity under his microscope. Some of the most prestigious medical doctors of the time, including Drs. E.C. Rosenow of the Mayo Clinic and Arthur Kendall of Northwestern University, also witnessed pleomorphic activity under the Rife microscope. (Other researchers in other times and places, most notably Guenther Enderlein, also came to discover on their own the truth of pleomorphism.)

There is reference in the internal minutes of the Mayo Clinic to the poliomyelitis virus having been viewed under the Rife microscope. And yet, today there is no library reference to Royal Rife, the man, his microscope, his work — nothing. It was totally obliterated until fairly recently. WHY? Why was his work suppressed? The WHY does not have so much to do with the microscope as it has to do with another of Rife's innovations — a frequency generator used for healing the body.

It had been Rife's goal in working with his microscope to identify the microorganism(s) associated with cancer, and he was successful toward that end. He identified four different forms of the micro-organism and found that it was only the *viral* form that caused tumors. But yet it was necessary to devitalize all of the other forms, as well, to successfully treat the disease. And, he went on to develop a means of effectively doing this by using a frequency generator. He successfully devitalized all forms of the cancer microorganism with radio wave frequencies. It is reported that Rife was curing terminal cancer patients by exposing them to specific frequencies for three minutes every third day. It is also said that he had cured 52 other diseases in like manner.

It was at this time, when he began working with the frequency generator, that things started to go wrong in Royal Rife's life. It was at this point that items began disappearing from his laboratory. His laboratory caught on fire, and he was brought into court on charges which were ultimately dismissed. All of these difficulties left Rife a broken man, financially and emotionally. He died virtually unknown in the 1970s. *The Cancer Cure That Worked* by Barry Lynes, released in 1987, is a comprehensive report of the Royal Rife story. Its publication triggered a resurgence of interest in Rife's work. Information regarding his work can now be accessed on line on the World Wide Web.

Intriguing as the work that Rife did with his frequency instrument is, the point I want to make about his work is that he gave us a tool by which we could *verify* the validity of pleomorphic activity. He gave us the microscope. While his work was suppressed, it was unknowingly carried on by a countryman of Béchamp, another Frenchman, who today lives and works in Canada. This man is Gaston Naessens. Naessens had never heard of the work of Antoine Béchamp. He had never heard of the work of Royal Rife. And yet, unknowingly, he merged the work of these two great men.

In 1949, working largely on his own, Gaston Naessens developed a light-source microscope capable of super-magnification that allowed the viewer to witness the activity of living microorganisms. In short, he developed a Rife-type microscope. Interestingly, his microscope was ineligible for patent because it defied the known laws of optics! Despite the fact that his microscope was not eligible for a patent, Gaston Naessens, using this remarkable instrument, went on, not only to verify, but to study, analyze and categorize pleomorphic activity. After many decades of study with this incredible microscope, Gaston Naessens came to some of the same basic conclusions Béchamp had come to 100 years earlier. Among those basic conclusions was that the stuff of which germs are made is our own genetic material. *The stuff of which germs are made is our own genetic material,* which is to say that disease is indeed "born in us and of us."[9] Germs, it seems, originate from an indestructible basic life particle that Béchamp called a microzyma and Naessens named a somatid.

Naessens came to believe that the electrically charged somatid is the original spark of life, the point in which energy condenses into matter.

Interestingly, at the end of 1999, there were absolutely no references to the work of Béchamp, Rife or Naessens found on the Internet under "Medline," the National Library of Medicine database. However, using the Yahoo search engine, references to all were found. This demonstrates that the work of these great men has yet to be acknowledged by the medical profession, though it is becoming known to the general public, to those willing to dig deep to find it.

To review the pleomorphic doctrine: According to it, disease is caused by (1) the *proliferation,* the multiplication of microbes or germs, and (2) by their *transformation* into virulent forms. The proliferation and transformation result from a shift in the terrain or context, the medium or internal environment of the host organism.

THE MICROBE IS NOTHING - THE TERRAIN IS EVERYTHING

It is significant that on his death bed, Louis Pasteur is said to have uttered these words: "Bernard was right, (Bernard was a proponent of the pleomorphic doctrine), *"the microbe is nothing, the terrain is everything."*(10) That death bed confession was a day late and a dollar short, for history went on to develop a huge medical monopoly based upon the false premise of monomorphic activity. According to the pleomorphic doctrine, anything that alters terrain causes disease by upsetting homeostasis. Homeostasis is the body's balancing mechanism, and balance is a key word in health. When the body is out of balance, energy can no longer flow freely. Energy blockages are set up, and that leads to disease conditions. Health, in a very real sense, is energy, energy flowing freely through the body without obstruction. Where there is imbalance, there is obstruction to energy flow (more on this in chapter 12). Therefore, it is very important that we get the body in balance and keep it in balance. Anything that adversely alters terrain also causes disease by producing conditions favorable to toxic build-up. When toxins build up in the body, then nature sends in her clean-up crew to take out the garbage. That clean-up crew is the altered forms of our own inherent germs.

So, according to the pleomorphic doctrine, germs do not cause disease. In fact, it might be said that disease causes germs. **Disease causes germs!** To fully understand that concept, imagine this scenario: Visualize, if you will, a stagnant pool of water around which mosquitoes are swarming. When you view this scene, do you conclude that the mosquitoes caused the water to become stagnant? Of course not! You know that it is the stagnant *conditions* in the water that draw the mosquitoes to it. Just as the polluted conditions in the pond draw mosquitoes to it, so, too, do polluted conditions in our bodies give rise to virulent forms of our own inherent germs. The natural healing perspective rests upon the validity of the pleomorphic doctrine which has been established and proven (though that proof has been buried). This doctrine emphasizes the *context* in which germs are found rather than the germs themselves. According to the pleomorphic doctrine, microorganisms *reflect* the conditions in which they are found. They do not *cause* those conditions. Therefore, in looking at the cause of disease from the natural healing perspective, we are not concerned with germs but rather with the context in which those germs are found, the **terrain.** It is, indeed, everything.

CONTEXTUAL FACTORS

There are many, many contextual factors that can move us in the direction of disease. Chief among them are:

- **Poor nutrition**
- **Malillumination** (poor lighting, a deficiency of light frequency)
- **Hypoventilation** (under breathing, shallow breathing)
- **Inactivity** (lack of exercise)
- **Electromagnetic pollution** (the effects of 60 cycle current, microwaves, etc.)
- **Environmental toxin**s (primarily man-made chemicals and heavy metals)
- **Negative thoughts/emotions**
- **Structural Imbalance**

All of these factors produce blockages and/or imbalance in the body, first in its subtle energy field and, ultimately, in the physical structure. All 8 factors are of equal importance. All interact and influence each other, contributing to the creation of disease. Each will be discussed, to one degree or another, in the pages that follow.

CB **CHAPTER 2** CB

Over-Consumption
Malnutrition

*"One third of what we eat keeps us alive. Two thirds
of what we eat keeps the doctors alive!"*
unknown

Americans are proud. We like to think of our nation as the greatest in the world — the wealthiest, the strongest and the healthiest. We certainly have the material wealth, and, if it could buy health, perhaps we'd have that too. It's not that we don't try. Our approximate two trillion dollar annual expenditure on health care exceeds that of any other nation. And yet, in terms of longevity, we fare very poorly. Our average life span is currently 71.6 years for men, 78.6 for women. This places us #16 in longevity among the nations of the world. The Japanese are #1, with males living an average of 76.2 years and females 82.5.[1]

There has been a dramatic increase in degenerative diseases in our country since the beginning of the 1900s. A major reason for this, and for our poor mortality rating, appears to be the prevalence of a condition that has been referred to as over-consumption malnutrition. OVER-CONSUMPTION MALNUTRITION: The American plague. What is it? It is, as its name implies, a condition wherein the body is malnourished while simultaneously being overfed.

We tend to think of malnourishment as resulting from undereating, but, in actuality, it is a consequence of taking too little nourishment into the system. The amount of nourishment a meal provides is not measured by the quantity of food but rather by the quality of it. We can eat tremendous quantities of food and still be malnourished (and therefore still hungry) when the quality of the food is substandard. Am I suggesting the Standard American Diet (SAD) may be substandard? Yes, I am! And moreover, I maintain that the SAD, composed of processed, refined, preserved, irradiated, enriched and otherwise devitalized food-like substances, is a root cause of the increase in degenerative diseases in our culture. And so, I postulate a cause-effect relationship that looks like this:

Intake of devitalized food

Condition of over-consumption malnutrition

Increase in degenerative disease

Let's look now at some of the factors responsible for this situation. On the top of the list, I would place:

THE ECONOMIC EXPEDIENCY OF MARKETING DEVITALIZED FOODS

Under this heading are included the practices of refining, enriching and preserving foods. The dictionary defines "refined" as (1) free from coarseness or vulgarity (2) free of impurities (3) precise to a fine degree; subtle, exact. All of these definitions have positive connotations which might lead one to believe that the refining process is a beneficial one. It is not. The food processors give a whole new dimension to the meaning of the word. The same may be said of "enriched." The name implies that the product has more or better ingredients than its unenriched counterpart. Not so again. These are misleading terms. Any refined food product has been altered from its natural state, subjected to a process that destroys much of its nutritional value. Unrefined is natural. Refined is not.

In 1862, machinery was invented that permitted milling of grains, giving them a lighter color, a finer texture — and a poorer nutrient content. The refining of grains involves the removal and disposal of their outer husks where most of the nutrients are concentrated. Wheat germ and bran, rice polish — these are removed during the milling process. Elimination of these nutritious parts of the grain from our diet has resulted in a widespread deficiency of B vitamins. Other vitamins and minerals, as well as fiber, are likewise lost. And the devitalized "enriched" product, such as white flour, acts quite literally like paste in the intestines (flour + water = paste. Remember that from grammar school?).

Lately, Americans have developed a fiber consciousness of sorts and consequently have purchased bran by the pound. The food processor is more than willing to increase his profits by packaging and marketing that portion of the grain formerly shipped off for animal feed. He profits twice, for the uninformed consumer purchases both the enriched grain product *and* a bag of bran to further enrich it, unaware that the grain in its natural state contained the bran until it was refined. Some of us are getting wise and purchasing the whole grain product instead. Some have even learned that fiber isn't found only in packages in grocery stores and in grains but richly abounds in fruits and vegetables.

During World War I, the milling of grains was forbidden in Denmark due to economic cutbacks. It is interesting to note that the death rate subsequently fell 34% ... during the war years! The incidence of cancer, kidney disease and diabetes (major degenerative diseases) also dropped markedly. Much the same thing happened in England during World War II when grains were only slightly milled.

White flour products are examples of refined grains. White rice is another example. When white rice took the world by storm and replaced its longer-cooking brown counterpart, there ensued the development of a dreaded disease named beriberi. About this time in history, the germ theory had gained widespread acceptance, and scientists were being offered incentives to find the "germ" responsible for causing the disease. They never did find it because beriberi is not caused by a germ but rather by a nutritional deficiency. This was discovered accidentally when sick animals were fed brown rice, rejected for human consumption, and became well. Thiamine or vitamin B1 is a component of the husk of brown rice. It is essential for the health of the nervous system. When the husks of the rice are discarded during the refining process, so is the B1, along with other B vitamins.

As time passed, it became embarrassingly obvious that the refining process destroyed vital nutrients. Enter the enriching process in 1941. Ever see one of those labels that reads something like "ENRICHED with vitamin B1, B2, niacin and iron?" Wow! — this means three B vitamins and one mineral (in their synthetic form) are added to a grain product that, before it was 'refined,' contained those nutrients in their natural form plus many, many more. So — the "enriching" process puts back a little — a very little — of what the refining process took out! The grain product is then about as enriched as you would be if someone stole $5000 from you and gave back $100. We can all think of more appropriate and accurate names than "enriched" for this process, but they wouldn't make for sound marketing strategy! Remember, anything that's enriched has first been impoverished.

There are currently more some 5000 additives in our food supply. This amounts to more than ten pounds of food additives — emulsifiers, stabilizers, thickeners, flavoring and coloring agents, preservatives, etc. consumed per person per year. Extending shelf life is the major reason for using food preservatives. And, indeed, shelf life *is* extended, for, as Adelle Davis pointed out in the 1960s in her classic, *Let's Eat Right to Keep Fit*, the preserved food "can't even support the health of bacteria, molds, weevils." Obviously it cannot support human health either.

The following exposé about additives used in ice cream appeared in the June 1958 edition of the magazine *Nature's Path:*

In the old days when ice cream was made of whole eggs, milk and sugar and laboriously cranked out in the old home freezer, a serving of ice cream was only an occasional family treat which didn't do much harm. Today, in this mass-producing, synthetic age, it is another matter entirely. Today, you may be "treating" your family to POISON.

Ice cream manufacturers are not required by law to list the additives used in the manufacture of their product. Consequently, today most ice creams are synthetic from start to finish. Analysis has shown the following:

DIETHYL GLUCOL - a cheap chemical used as an emulsifier instead of eggs; the same chemical used in antifreeze and in paint removers.

PIPERONAL - used in place of vanilla. This is a chemical used to kill lice.

ALDEHYDE C 17 - used to flavor cherry ice cream. It is an inflammable liquid which is also used in aniline dyes, plastic and rubber.

ETHYL ACETATE - used to give ice cream a pineapple flavor. It is also used as a cleaner for leather and textiles, and its vapors have been known to cause chronic lung, liver and heart damage.

BUTYRALDEHYDE - used in nut flavored ice cream. It's one of the ingredients in rubber cement.

AMYL ACETATE - used for its banana flavor. It's also used as an oil paint solvent.

BENZYL ACETATE - used for its strawberry flavor. It's a nitrate solvent.

So -- the next time you're tempted by a luscious looking banana split sundae, think of it as a mixture of antifreeze, oil paint, nitrate solvent and lice killer, and you won't find it so appetizing!

Too few of us bother to read ingredients on labels. There's an art to it. Or perhaps it's more of a science. A background in chemistry would certainly be helpful in deciphering many a label, replete as they tend to be with chemical jargon. A good rule of thumb is this: If the list of ingredients is lengthy and the words hard to pronounce, don't buy it! It's useful to know that ingredients are listed in descending order in terms of quantity present in the food. For example, if sugar is the #1 ingredient (as it so often is), there's more of it than anything else in the food. If the last ingredient listed is salt, there's less salt (though there still may be a considerable amount of it) than any other ingredient.

Lest we worry over much about the possible damage caused by the 5000 or so additives in our food supply, the government offers new hope, an alternative to chemical preservatives or at least a method that will help (they say) decrease their use and still prolong shelf life:

FOOD IRRADIATION

Food irradiation, the process of zapping food with nuclear radiation for the purpose of preserving it, isn't really new. It was first patented in the 1930s by French scientists. Thirty years later, it was approved by the FDA for use on wheat and potatoes. The process was not taken too seriously at that time, however, as cheaper chemical methods of preservation were preferred. By the mid-1980s, a fresh look was taken at food irradiation after EDB (ethylene dibromide), a widely used chemical fumigant, was banned. By 1986, the irradiation of herbs and spices was approved at a dose of up to 3 million RADS (Radiation Absorbed Doses) — the equivalent of *2 million chest x-rays!* Since then, the government has granted approval of irradiation of virtually all foods, using even higher doses, despite the fact that their own evidence indicates that the process results in creation of "carcinogens, mutagens and other potential toxins."[2]

While the federal government claims the absolute safety of the food irradiation process, the fact of the matter is that FDA approval was not based on tests demonstrating its safety but rather upon the theoretical estimate of the number of Unique Radiolytic Products (URPs) likely to result from the process. To understand what this means, we must first know that gamma rays, with their ionizing effect, have the ability to knock electrons out of atoms. Ionizing radiation gives rise to the creation of free radicals, renegade chemical fragments that have been demonstrated to play a significant role in the aging and degenerative disease processes. The free radical is a molecule with an unpaired electron of either a positive or negative charge. A URP is formed when two of these chemical fragments of unlike charge unite. A myriad of possible combinations are created, with the possibility of some of the newly created URPs being carcinogenic. Radiolytic products include formaldehyde, benzene, formic acid and quinones, all of which are quite toxic.

As far as studies go, the first food irradiation research done in this country was in the 1950s on canned bacon in the army. The 1963 FDA clearance of the use of the irradiated product was withdrawn in 1968 due to the discovery that the research was flawed. Much of the research supporting food irradiation was carried out by Industrial Biotest Limited. In 1983, three of their officials were convicted for fraudulent research for government and industry.[3] And yet the federal government assures us that studies indicate that the process is safe. What studies? Surely not the ones conducted in 1975 on Indian children who showed blood changes similar to leukemia three weeks after consuming freshly irradiated wheat? Surely not those studies that prompted Germany and other countries to ban food irradiation? Harvey Diamond tells us that "an internal 1982 FDA audit showed that only 1% of 413 studies conducted over 30 years appeared to support safety [of the process]."[4]

Ill-effects cited by German scientists included mutations, decreased growth rate, reduced resistance to disease, changes in organ weight and development of tumors. Kidney damage has also resulted from the irradiation process. It should also be pointed out that nutrients are destroyed or modified by the ionizing effect of irradiation. An estimated 20-80% of nutrients, including vitamins A, B, C, E and K, as well as the essential fatty acids and amino acids, are thus affected. With this kind of nutrient loss from irradiation, further loss during storage and even further nutrient depletion with cooking, with what are we left? We're left with dangerously devitalized food.

Proponents of food irradiation point out that it destroys bacteria.

It should be noted, however, that even if bacteria are killed, toxins created by the bacteria at earlier stages of contamination are not removed. It is observed also that irradiation at approved levels slows the ripening of fruits and vegetables but is not high enough to destroy such microorganisms as botulism. The smell, however, *is* eradicated, increasing the danger of inadvertent consumption of contaminated food. Another concern is the probable proliferation of toxic, radiation-resistant microorganisms.

Over the years, Food and Water, Inc. has done much to educate the public about the adverse effects of the irradiation process. Their success led them to tackle other issues — the use of Bovine Growth Hormone and pesticides in agriculture. More on these later.

Food and Water's early success with the food irradiation issue is reflected in public opinion polls which indicate the unpopularity of the process. In a 1994 Health Focus Survey, 82% of American consumers indicated they were concerned about food irradiation. Food and Water has also been instrumental in turning food manufacturers away from irradiation. Since 1986, one hundred food corporations have pledged not to use irradiation on their food. Quaker Oaks, H.J. Heinz and Ralston Purina are among those who have stopped irradiating. It is also encouraging that Florida's Food Technology Services (formerly Vindicator), the nation's first irradiation facility, lost nearly 5 million dollars during its first four years of operation. This facility, like other early ones in this country, employs gamma source irradiators which infuse foods with cobalt-60, a radioactive isotope. Cesium 137, a by-product of plutonium (used for nuclear warhead production) extraction, has also been used.

Due to the unpopularity of food irradiation as it was originally practiced, the process has been given a new look — and may be getting a new name (the benign-sounding "cold pasteurization" has been proposed). In an effort to get the public to accept food irradiation, the U.S. government has worked diligently to diminish labeling requirements, push through new irradiation approvals and obtain funding for marketing and "consumer education." They have been largely successful. The 1997 Modernization Act eliminated the requirement that the radura (stylized flower symbol) be present on the label of irradiated foods. It stated that disclosure information regarding irradiation need be "no more prominent than required for the declaration of ingredients." Government spokesmen have made the following false/unsubstantiated claims and absurd recommendations regarding food irradiation:

(1) Radiation-treated foods posed "no toxicological" risks for consumers (FDA claim, endorsed by the USDA).

(2) Irradiated food products would be ideal for the school lunch program...[with]...no need for any special notification of the parents of children participating. (USDA).

(3) Irradiators have been shown to operate without significant radiation risk to workers or the public. (USDA)(5)

This last statement totally ignores documented cases of ground water contamination, injury and loss of lives caused by irradiation accidents over the years.

The 'new look' that food irradiation has taken on incorporates the use of electron beams or high energy lasers. A new leader has emerged in the construction of irradiation facilities. — Titan Corporation of San Diego, California. A military contractor, Titan was developer of the "Star Wars" missile defense system laser technology. This company plans construction of irradiation facilities in Hawaii (for exportation of tropical fruits), in Iowa (for red meat) and in Arkansas (for poultry and other meats).

Alarmingly, Titan has a growing number of food industry supporters, including IBP and Cargill (top meat corporations in the U.S.) and Tyson Foods (leading poultry producer). A new organization, the Food Irradiation Coalition, comprised of 30+ major food associations, has been instrumental in paving the way for public acceptance of the food irradiation process.

Despite the public's continual opposition to food irradiation, its proponents persist in promoting it heavily and lobbying for its acceptance. As Food and Water, Inc. warns, "Unless we act now, some day it may be difficult to find non-irradiated foods"... You can take action by joining Food and Water in their grass roots campaigns against the tainting of our food and water supplies. Contact them at 1-800-EAT-SAFE (www.foodandwater.org) to request an information packet.

It is plain to see, on the basis of the foregoing data, how vested financial interest within the food industry, with its practices of "refinement," "enrichment," chemical preservation and food irradiation, is making a huge contribution to the devitalization and contamination of our food supply and thus to the condition of over-consumption malnutrition. A question that logically follows is, "How can this be happening; how can we *allow* this to happen?" Unfortunately, due largely to overwhelmingly successful advertising efforts, Americans are not only allowing, but are now demanding the production and delivery of fast foods, junk foods, non-food foods. A major reason for this is seen as:

LACK OF EDUCATION

I speak here not only of the lack of education of the general public but also a deficiency of education within the medical profession. Only about 1/3 of our medical schools offer courses in nutrition, and only half of those make enrollment in them mandatory. What little nutrition education *is* offered, both in medical schools and in other institutions of learning, has been based, for the most part, on the well-known, but outdated and inaccurate "Four Food Groups" or the newer food pyramid. There are inherent flaws in both of these models as we'll see shortly.

As the late Dr. Robert Mendelsohn, M.D., repeatedly pointed out, the "Church of Modern Medicine" is the religion of the masses in the U.S. The word "doctor" is synonymous with medical doctor in the minds of most. We have been very thoroughly indoctrinated to believe that allopathic medicine (the chemically oriented kind we know so well) is the only valid system of health care. We're led to believe that other systems are "unscientific quackery," and we're cautioned to "Beware of the Health Hucksters" (title of an old *Readers Digest* article) who offer "dangerous" alternatives. One cannot help but wonder what is endangered — the health of the people or the reign of the medical monopoly?

The truth of the matter is that, contrary to AMA propaganda, the medical doctor is not the only type of physician practicing in this country, nor is s/he the only type who is qualified, competent and licensed. Three other types of physicians are trained and licensed in the U.S. at present: chiropractors (D.C.s), osteopaths (D.O.s)

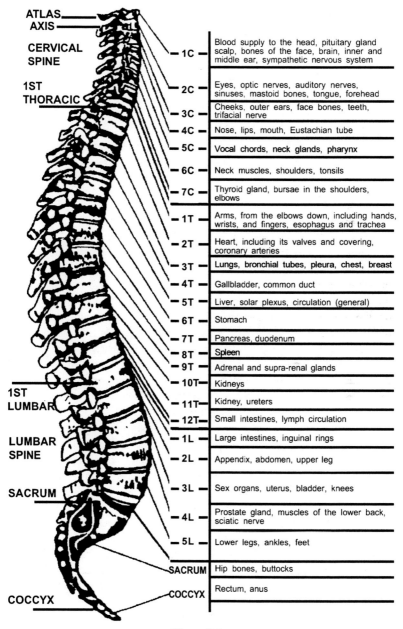

ATLAS
AXIS

CERVICAL SPINE

1ST THORACIC

1ST LUMBAR

LUMBAR SPINE

SACRUM

COCCYX

1C	Blood supply to the head, pituitary gland scalp, bones of the face, brain, inner and middle ear, sympathetic nervous system
2C	Eyes, optic nerves, auditory nerves, sinuses, mastoid bones, tongue, forehead
3C	Cheeks, outer ears, face bones, teeth, trifacial nerve
4C	Nose, lips, mouth, Eustachian tube
5C	Vocal chords, neck glands, pharynx
6C	Neck muscles, shoulders, tonsils
7C	Thyroid gland, bursae in the shoulders, elbows
1T	Arms, from the elbows down, including hands, wrists, and fingers, esophagus and trachea
2T	Heart, including its valves and covering, coronary arteries
3T	Lungs, bronchial tubes, pleura, chest, breast
4T	Gallbladder, common duct
5T	Liver, solar plexus, circulation (general)
6T	Stomach
7T	Pancreas, duodenum
8T	Spleen
9T	Adrenal and supra-renal glands
10T	Kidneys
11T	Kidney, ureters
12T	Small intestines, lymph circulation
1L	Large intestines, inguinal rings
2L	Appendix, abdomen, upper leg
3L	Sex organs, uterus, bladder, knees
4L	Prostate gland, muscles of the lower back, sciatic nerve
5L	Lower legs, ankles, feet
SACRUM	Hip bones, buttocks
COCCYX	Rectum, anus

Chart 2A

and naturopaths (N.D.s). Let's take a brief look at each of these professions:

CHIROPRACTIC

Chiropractic, as an organized system of health care, was developed by D.D. Palmer in 1895. It is based on the theory that disease is due primarily to impingement of nerves. As the spinal chart (2A) shows, the spine is divided into three segments: cervical (neck), thoracic (mid back) and lumbar (lower back). Between each vertebra or large bone in these segments, spinal nerves are interlaced. These nerves all lead to specific areas of the body. For example, note that T-10 (the tenth thoracic vertebra) leads to the kidneys. If a patient is suffering from a kidney disorder, the doctor of chiropractic would most certainly be interested in the positioning of T-10. If it is "subluxated" or misaligned, it would be exerting pressure or impinging upon the tenth thoracic nerve which supplies nerve energy to the kidneys. That organ then would be hampered in its ability to receive nerve impulses. Circulation, too, would be impaired, with lack of nutrients and oxygen to the kidney area. By re-seating the vertebrae into their correct positions (at the level of T-10 and elsewhere), proper nerve supply and circulation are restored to the kidneys and other organs, and the body then has the energy available to it to mobilize its own healing resources. The re-seating of misaligned vertebrae by a doctor of chiropractic is known as a chiropractic adjustment and may be accomplished manually (in which case a 'pop' is often heard or felt as the vertebra goes back into position). Gentler chiropractic adjustments may be made with the aid of instruments which lightly 'tap' the vertebra back into position.

Chiropractors are typically thought of as treating only back problems because they concentrate on the spine. This is not so. Because spinal nerves supply energy to the entire body, spinal adjustments can affect all parts of it. The bony structures are adjusted to affect changes in the nervous system. The range of disorders that can be treated by chiropractic is very wide, for it is an entire system of health care, albeit a nonmedical one.

Many of us have been taught to think of chiropractors as "quacks." It has not been a profession that has enjoyed a great deal of respect until relatively recently. Why? Is it because of lack of training of the chiropractor? Or a lack of efficacy of his/her techniques? Neither. Amazingly, many of our misconceptions about chiropractors came from the American Medical Association. On 8/27/87, Federal Judge, Susan Getzendanner, found the AMA, along with the American College of Surgeons and the American College of Radiologists, guilty of conspiring to destroy the chiropractic profession. It was established in the 11-year trial that the AMA paid a team of over a dozen M.D.s, attorneys and others to attempt to destroy the chiropractic profession in this country. This was done with the full knowledge and support of the executive officers of the AMA. AMA agents dispersed throughout the country referred to chiropractors as "rabid dogs," "killers," "cultists," "unscientific" and "quacks." These are the actual terms that showed up in AMA documents. On 2/7/90, the U.S. Court of Appeals for the Seventh Circuit upheld the guilt of the AMA, the judge stating that they had acted unlawfully, "violating the antitrust laws by conspiring with its members and other medical professional societies to destroy the profession of chiropractic in the United States." Clearly the AMA has done much to damage the chiropractic profession. Let's look at some of the facts about this health care system and the training of their physicians. The chart on page 30 compares the education of a D.C. to that of a M.D.

This data was compiled from a review of the curriculum of 22 medical schools and 11 chiropractic colleges and updated from the *National Health Federation Bulletin* and other publications' statistics. We can see that the chiropractic student takes more hours of anatomy, physiology, bacteriology, diagnosis, neurology, x-ray and orthopedics than does the medical student. This might explain why chiropractors were found (according to testimony given in the trial) to be *twice* as effective as medical doctors in treating musculoskeletal problems.

Many chiropractic colleges require courses in nutrition. While the D.C. can, and frequently does, utilize and dispense nutritional supplements, s/he cannot prescribe drugs nor perform surgery. Such practices are outside the realm of not only his/her expertise, but also outside of the philosophy of the profession. At present, chiropractors do not generally have hospital privileges.

Today, despite AMA attempts at suppression, chiropractors are licensed in every state and their services covered by insurance.

The profession is gaining much earned respect despite the many obstacles placed before it by the AMA.

MEDICAL Class Hours (minimum)	Subject	CHIROPRACTIC Class Hours (minimum)
508	Anatomy	520
326	Physiology	420
401	Pathology	205
325	Chemistry	300
114	Bacteriology	130
324	Diagnosis	420
112	Neurology	320
148	X-ray	217
144	Psychiatry	65
198	Obstetrics & GYN	65
156	Orthopedics	225
2,756	TOTAL HOURS	2,887

Other required subjects for the Doctor of Chiropractic: adjusting, manipulation, kinesiology and other similar basic subjects related to his specialty. Other required subjects for the Doctor of Medicine: pharmacology, immunology, general surgery and other similar basic subjects related to his specialty.

GRAND TOTAL CLASS HOURS Including Other Basic Subjects		
4,248		**4,485**

OSTEOPATHY

It was a M.D., Andrew Still, who was credited with developing osteopathy in 1874. Osteopathy is based on the theory that sickness is due to sluggishness of the vital body functions. The traditional D.O. therefore practices bodily manipulation (much like chiropractic adjustment) to stimulate the circulation of blood and lymph. Dr. Still, though a licensed M.D., insisted that the body needed no drugs. This is the philosophy of traditional osteopathy. However, somewhere along the way, medical practices became intermingled with osteopathic ones. Today, osteopaths throughout the country are licensed to practice medicine, including surgery and the prescription of drugs. Certain colleges in the United States are accredited by the American Osteopathic Association to offer the required four-year course of training and grant the D.O. degree. These colleges also give complete instruction in conventional medicine. The typical osteopath in practice today has, however, abandoned clinical use of the manipulation skills learned in school and is thus indistinguishable from his/her medical counterpart. Every now and then, we may encounter an "old school" osteopath who still practices manipulation, but s/he is (sadly) the exception and not the rule.

NATUROPATHY

The term "naturopathy" was coined by John H. Scheel in 1895, but the profession was given its biggest boost by Benedict Lust who came to the U.S. from Germany to introduce the Kneipp water cures. This remarkable man was a M.D., a D.O. and a N.D. He founded the American Naturopathic Society in 1919.

The naturopath is probably the most versatile of the physicians, for s/he is trained in all forms of natural healing. We can expect the naturopathic physician to have some knowledge of a variety of treatment and diagnostic modalities, which may include bodily adjustments and manipulations, herbology, homeopathy, iridology, acupuncture, nutrition, etc. The D.C. may choose to study and become certified in any of these areas too, but, except for adjustment and manipulation, these subjects are not emphasized in his formal training. In theory, the M.D. or D.O. may also become certified in any of these areas. In practice, however, he rarely does, for they are not likely to appeal to him (having a different philosophical orientation than medicine). And, were he to practice them, he would risk being ostracized by members of his own profession.

Naturopathy was a well-respected profession that gained in popularity for another decade or so after the American Naturopathy Society was founded by Dr. Lust. It was the introduction of the "wonder drugs" (antibiotics) and the widespread acceptance of the germ theory that caused naturopathy to drop in popularity.

Today naturopathy, like chiropractic, is struggling to regain acceptance and is meeting with some success, though it has not made the strides that chiropractic has in the nation as a whole. A growing number of states are licensing naturopathic physicians.

If chiropractic, traditional osteopathy and naturopathy, as described above, really are valid alternatives to medicine, why are so many unaware of this? The answer takes us back once again in time:

In the early 1900s, the Rockefeller and Carnegie Foundations became quite heavily involved in the practice of giving philanthropic grants to medical schools. Their goal was to create an exclusively male, upper class medical profession rooted in the philosophy of allopathic medicine or drug therapy. In 1909, they sent a man named Abraham Flexner on a tour of all schools involved in health care training. The following year, the Flexner Report was issued. After that, the number of medical degree-granting institutions in the U.S. dropped from approximately 400 down to 65. By reducing the number of medical physicians, supply went down, and demand increased. The medical doctor began building a monopoly over the delivery of health care in the U.S. The Flexner Report dealt a severe blow to all nonmedical health care systems, for the Rockefellers and Carnegies, with their legislative clout, were influential in having regulations passed which limited official recognition to the medical approach. The Rockefellers were heavily vested in the pharmaceutical industry.

Apart from the legislative domain, the credibility of medicine is suffering as a consequence of its own failures. Medicine is concerned with the study of disease and suppression of symptoms. As previously discussed, such suppression can actually be dangerous to the patient. The suppression of disease symptoms through the use of allopathic medicine does not remove the basic cause of the problem but does, in fact, exacerbate it by driving toxins deeper into the tissues of the body. The average hospital patient today is given six different drugs. With six different drugs, there is a 100% chance of adverse interaction and the development of serious side effects. This is the stuff of which iatrogenic disease is made. The medical profession stands in violation of its first law: DO NO HARM.

THE BASIC FOUR

Apart from the harm done by medicine, we do much harm to ourselves when we consume the SAD (Standard American Diet). Even the "good nutrition" models taught in our schools can lead us to poor health.

Most of us were raised on the notion of the four food groups mentioned earlier. We were taught that, in order to be healthy, it was necessary to eat from each of these groups daily.

Let's look at the four food groups from the point of view of the effect they have on the terrain of the body in terms of pH. PH is measurement of acidity/alkalinity. In the first group, we have meat, an acid-forming food. Acid-*forming* means that once it has been metabolized, it leaves an acid ash in the body. The second group, dairy, is also acid-forming, if we are talking about *commercial* cow milk products. They leave an acid ash once metabolized, as does the third group, grains. All grains, with the exception of millet (and possibly buckwheat), also leave an acid ash in the body. The only one of the traditional four food groups that does not leave an acid ash is the fruit and vegetable group. This is the only one of the groups that is alkaline-forming.

So, you can see that if we were to take seriously the advice about the four food groups and ate equally from each of these every day, we would be consuming a diet that is 3/4 or 75% acid-forming, since three of the four food groups contain food that is acid-forming. This is just the opposite of what we now know a good health-promoting diet would be, about 75 to 80% alkaline-forming. In other words, we want the majority of our foods to come from the fruit and vegetable group. If we do not take in enough alkaline-forming food in our diet; that is, enough fruits and vegetables, then we will deplete our alkaline reserves and be unable to deal with stress or illness. And this is exactly what is happening today.

The SAD is very over-acid. It is over-acid because it is made up primarily of foods other than fruits and vegetables. I'll have more to say about acid/alkaline balance in the next chapter, but for now, my point is this: The four food group concept that was taught as gospel for several decades is not based on sound nutrition; it's not based on scientific principles. What it *is* based on is vested interest, for it was the Kellogg people (of Corn Flake fame) who first came up with the idea of the four food groups. And they were later joined by the meat people and the dairy people. And it became for us an accepted truth — this commercial message. It has been suggested that the four food groups might more accurately have been called the four food *lobbies!*

THE NEW FOOD PYRAMID

Over the years, those who have been knowledgeable in the field of nutrition opposed vigorously the concept of the four food groups and sought to replace it with something more accurate. The first almost-successful effort to replace the four food group model with an alternative one occurred in April 1991, when the Physician's Committee for Responsible Medicine, headed by four respected, nutritionally oriented medical doctors, formally proposed a "New Four Foods Groups" to the U.S. Dept. of Agriculture. This new four foods group was made up of (1) vegetables (2) fruits (3) legumes (peas, beans, lentils) and (4) whole grains. Conspicuously absent from the model was meat and dairy. This was upsetting to you-know-who. Due to extensive lobbying on behalf of the meat and dairy industries, this proposal was defeated. One year later, in April, 1992, the new Food Pyramid was adopted. It looks like this:

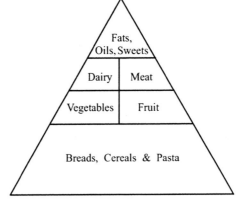

This pyramid is divided into four quadrants. The bottom quadrant consists of grains, and the advice is that we eat 6-11 servings daily. The next quadrant up is shared by fruits and vegetables.

The advice here is to eat 5 servings of vegetables and 2-4 servings of fruit daily. Meat and dairy are back in the picture in the third tier from the bottom, and we are advised to eat from 2 to 3 servings of each of these. At the very top of the pyramid are fats, oils and sweets, which we are told to "use sparingly."

The message that the food pyramid is actually *supposed to* convey is that we should be eating more of the foods at the bottom of the pyramid, those forming the base; that is, the grains and the foods directly above it, the fruits and vegetables. However, the pyramid is a very deceiving configuration, for when one looks at the pyramid shape, where does the eye go first? It goes to the apex. It goes to the top of the pyramid, and, what is at the top of the pyramid? Oils and sweets! So, subliminally, when we look at the food pyramid, the message we are getting is to "eat sweets." "Eat sweets and eat fats" — and that is just what Americans have been doing: eating sweets, eating fat and *getting* fat. When you look at the food pyramid from this point of view, meat and dairy are not only back in the picture, but they are back in a very prominent position, near the top. Being at the top has long been associated with being best. So, the new food pyramid, by putting oils and sweets at the very top (where the eye goes first), and dairy and meat in the second place, actually gives them an elevated status. Now, I have no argument with meat and dairy products, as long as they are good-quality meat and dairy products and as long as they are used in moderation. The problem, however, with meat and dairy products in our culture is that they are heavily processed, contaminated and overused. More on this in chapter 11.

A NEW DIETARY PARADIGM

The food pyramid, as a replacement for the four traditional food groups, is a step in the right direction. Its message is that we should build our diet on a foundation of starchy carbohydrates. It is very possible that by recommending up to 11 servings per day of carbohydrates, not distinguishing between refined and unrefined foods, and by placing sweets in a prominent position in the chart, the food pyramid may be encouraging or condoning the over-consumption of refined carbohydrates.

The food pyramid is a visual representation of the dietary paradigm (model) that has dominated our culture's consciousness for the last two decades. That paradigm tells us that a high carbohydrate/low fat diet is the ideal to which we should aspire to achieve weight loss, good health and peak performance. Even we "health nuts" have bought into this paradigm, for many alternative eating regimens feature meals even higher in carbs (albeit complex ones) and lower in fat than the SAD. The evidence is mounting that we've been dead wrong.

America's love affair with the high carbohydrate/low fat diet has ironically resulted in widespread weight gain and an increased incidence of degenerative disease. I first became aware of this several years ago when I was doing research for *Super Nutrition for Men*, the book I wrote in conjunction with Ann Louise Gittleman. The bulk of the research I reviewed for the book had been done by a then-unheard-of research scientist named Barry Sears. Dr. Sears has since come out with his own best-selling books on the subject, written in layman's language.

The bottom line is that our beloved high carbohydrate/low fat diet causes hormonal imbalances by promoting almost continuous insulin response (triggered by eating carbs) and inhibiting glucagon release (triggered by protein consumption). This results in fat storage (getting fat!) and lowering of blood sugar. Insulin/glucagon imbalance caused by consumption of too much carbohydrate in relation to protein, coupled with deficiencies of essential fatty acids due to inadequate intake of healthy fats, results in production of bad *eicosanoids*. Eicosanoids are obscure, but vitally important hormones that regulate virtually all body systems, especially the cardiovascular system. Food choices determine whether "good" or "bad" eicosanoids will be produced.

Theoretically, by decreasing carbohydrate consumption (to 40% of calories in the diet) and assuring an adequate intake of good quality, useable protein (30% of the diet) and natural, unprocessed fats (30%), we can lose weight effortlessly, regulate blood sugar levels and normalize eicosanoid production, favorably affecting all organs and systems in the body.

I became curious about Sears' 40/30/30 eating plan while working on *Super Nutrition for Men*. My curiosity increased after reading his book, *Enter the Zone*, but I never put it to the test because it did not seem to be very "user friendly" and appeared to overlook some important nutritional facts. I did, however, adopt a somewhat similar eating plan, one that features reduced consumption of starchy carbohydrates, called the *Pro Vita Plan,* several years ago and have stuck with it. I chose this plan because it made sense, is easy to implement — and it works. Its creator, the late Stuart Wheelwright, had a superior understanding of not only the chemistry of nutrition but the *energetic* properties of food. You can read about the details of Wheelwright's work and the *Pro Vita Plan* in a book by that title written by Jack Tips, N.D., Ph.D. I'll have more to say about it later as well.

BOTTOM LINE

The bottom line is that our official model of "good nutrition," the food pyramid, promotes and perpetuates the myth of the high carbohydrate diet as a superior one. It fails to distinguish between whole foods and processed, devitalized ones and thus promotes imbalanced eating.

Mineral depletion of our soils (discussed in the next chapter), food processing, food irradiation — are all factors that contribute to a nutrient-depleted food supply and to the epidemic of over-consumption malnutrition. The widespread use of chemicals in agriculture has increased the toxicity of both our food supply and the environment. With both toxicity and deficiency on the increase, so is degenerative disease.

CHAPTER 3

Disease Causation

"So long as one feeds on food from unhealthy soil, the spirit will lack the stamina to free itself from the prison of the body."
Rudolph Steiner

Dr. Harold Reilly in *The Edgar Cayce Handbook for Health Through Drugless Therapy* speaks about "C.A.R.E."(Circulation, Assimilation, Relaxation and Elimination). If the body is functioning normally in all of these areas, the result is good health. However, if there is impairment in any one of these processes, others will be affected, and ill health results, whether or not it manifests in diagnosed disease or even expresses as overt symptoms. Let's look at each component in Dr. Reilly's C.A.R.E. model:

CIRCULATION

Circulation refers to the movement of blood and lymph fluid through the body. The lymphatic system is the lifeline of the immune system and is discussed more fully in the next chapter. Circulation of blood provides the oxygen essential for metabolic processes and also removes carbon dioxide, formed as a waste product. Most of us believe that the oxygen we breathe in is exhaled as carbon dioxide. Actually, the oxygen unites with hydrogen in the body and is excreted as water through the kidneys. Carbon dioxide is the acid residue produced by normal metabolic processes. We do excrete it, in part, through our exhalations. Acid from foods is eliminated primarily through the kidneys after being neutralized.

The heart is the amazing pump that keeps our blood circulating. Each day it beats 100,000 times and pumps 4300 gallons of blood. Circulatory problems can result in stroke, heart attack, atherosclerosis (hardening of the arteries) and senility (decreased blood supply to the brain). Since the blood carries oxygen and nutrients to all the cells, impairment in circulation to a given organ or area of the body will result in energy loss at that site. To stimulate circulation, it is helpful to engage regularly in some form of aerobic exercise. Use of a rebounder (mini-trampoline) is especially stimulating to lymphatic circulation, as is use of a "Chi" machine, which provides a passive form of aerobic exercise. Massage, manipulation and the practice of "dry brushing" the skin also stimulate circulation. A natural bristle, long handled brush is used for dry brushing. The body is brushed vigorously in an upward motion toward the heart from the extremities. This is well to do once or twice daily. A good time is just before showering, for the brushing also removes particles of dead skin. In this manner, the eliminatory function of the skin is assisted.

The flow of blood to the brain is critically important, for interruption of it for just a few minutes can result in a coma; a few more minutes and permanent brain damage is done. Unimpaired circulation is vital to our health and well being.

ASSIMILATION

Assimilation is the individual's capacity to utilize food. This is a critical function, for even the best of foods will not nourish us if we cannot assimilate, or utilize, the nutrients from it. Assimilation includes absorption, the process by which nutrients are taken up by the intestines and passed into the bloodstream, as well as the digestive process.

Our ability to assimilate food is largely dependent upon the other three processes in the C.A.R.E. model. Increased circulation will aid in the absorption of nutrients. Thorough elimination is also essential, for incomplete elimination will block nutrient absorption in the intestines and result in lack of nourishment to the rest of the body. Likewise, relaxation permits assimilation, while the stress response inhibits it. When the pH of the body is off, assimilation is hampered. PH is largely regulated through diet.

RELAXATION

If we're going to digest our food, it is essential that the body be in a relaxed state at meal time. Unfortunately, most of us are used to eating on the go and rushing our meals. We learned this at lunch time when we were kids in school. It was often a wait to get through the line in the cafeteria, then a race to consume the food in the allotted half hour. Then we grew up, went to work and got an hour for lunch (some of us), but we're still rushed, for most of us find numerous other activities to cram into our lunch hour. Even if the hour *is* devoted to eating, it still may be stressful, for many a business deal is consummated at meal time. Sadly, we are not taught to take our time, sit in silence and savor our food. Meal time is, unfortunately, too often social time, and the topics and pace of conversation can be most upsetting to the digestion. Rushed as we are, we do not take the time to thoroughly masticate our food — a few gnashes of the teeth, and it's swallowed practically whole, never to be digested, for the process of digestion begins in the mouth, with the secretion of digestive juices. Practitioners of macrobiotics (a Japanese system of living and eating) teach that we should chew each mouthful of food *fifty times* before swallowing it! Try it sometime — even thirty times would be an effort for most of us.

The condition of our mind and emotions at meal time is extremely important. If we eat when we're tired, angry, excited or under stress, we'll develop indigestion. If we make a habit of it, an ulcer can result.

A relaxed state is facilitated by correct breathing. Deep abdominal breathing relaxes the mind and body and provides oxygen to the tissues. Most of us breathe in a shallow manner from the chest. This habitual aberrant pattern is conducive to a build-up of stress in the system. More information on breathing is given in the next chapter.

The body's reactions to stress include (1) rise in blood pressure (2) rise in blood sugar (3) increase in stomach acid (4) constriction of the arteries and (5) shrinkage of the thymus gland. Most of us are familiar with the consequences of the first four effects, but what about the thymus? During the stress response, compounds are released by the adrenal gland that cause this gland to shrink. To understand the significance of this effect, we need to take a closer look at the thymus gland.

THE THYMUS GLAND

Our thymus gland is located about an inch beneath the notch where the clavicles come together at the center of the upper chest, just below the neck (where the second rib joins the breastbone). This gland is what is known as "sweetbread" in calves.

For a long time, the standard medical teaching was that the thymus gland has NO FUNCTION. This conclusion was based largely on the fact that autopsies repeatedly showed the gland to be shrunken or atrophied.

In the 1950s, it was learned that, not only does the thymus gland have a function, it plays a critically important role in the functioning of the immune system. Helper T cells (a form of white blood cell described more fully in the next chapter) mature in the thymus and settle in lymph nodes and cells there. It is the release of the thymus hormone that activates these T cells in the immune response. Without release of this hormone, abnormal cells may not be recognized by the body, and diseases such as cancer will spread unchecked, for T cell function (activating the body's defenses) is impaired. The health of the thymus gland is imperative to insure the release of its hormone to trigger the immune response. When pre-1950s autopsies consistently showed shrunken thymus glands, the reason was a mystery.

The thymus plays an active role in the growth process but diminishes in size after puberty when the bulk of growing is done. It has been found that *further shrinkage is due to stress*. Under acute stress, the gland can shrink to half its size within 24 hours. This may happen as a consequence of severe injury or sudden illness. This finding sheds new light on the reason why post mortems consistently revealed shrunken thymus glands. But the effects of stress on the gland were unknown in the first half of the 20th century, and when it was discovered that babies who had died of the so-called "crib death" (SIDS) had enlarged thymus glands, it was mistakenly concluded that this thymus enlargement was the cause of death. A new disease was thus created: STATUS THYMICOLYMPHATICUS, and in the 1920s, 30s and 40s, children with enlarged thymus glands were treated with irradiation to "cure" the disorder by shrinking the gland! Whatever effect this may have had upon those children's presenting symptoms, we can be certain that it also gravely damaged their immune systems, making them more susceptible to all manner of infectious disease. Such diseases would be examples of iatrogenic disorders.

The fact that most of us have underactive thymus glands can be demonstrated by a simple muscle test. Put one hand over the thymus area and extend the other (thumb down) straight out. Test the muscle on that arm by having someone apply gentle, steady pressure, pushing the hand downward as you resist. If you cannot resist the pressure when your other hand is over the thymus, but can resist it when the thymus is uncovered, that is an indicator that the energy supply to the gland is reduced. To temporarily increase the energy flow, thump gently on the thymus area with your fists. Make like Tarzan. You should now find your test muscle is strong when you cover the thymus with the other hand. For more on this subject, look into *Your Body Doesn't Lie* by psychiatrist Dr. John Diamond.

The power of relaxation to heal is demonstrated through the success of biofeedback. Through this process, which conditions a person to relax, it has been found that control can be gained over autonomic functions previously thought not to be influenced by conscious thought. People have successfully controlled their blood pressure and diminished and eliminated migraine headaches through biofeedback. Meditation has also been shown to reverse stress reactions.

The power of the mind to heal is becoming increasingly acknowledged. Dr. Carl Simonton has had impressive results in treating cancer patients by teaching them to visualize the healing process. The late Norman Cousins, in his book *Anatomy of an Illness*, highlights the importance of humor and a positive outlook in victory over disease. Faced with an "incurable" disease, Cousins decided not to let his poor prognosis influence his expectation of recovery. He took responsibility for his health and laughed through the pain, even having Marx Brothers movies brought into his hospital room. This attitude was a significant factor in his recovery, though admittedly nutrition played an important role also.

ELIMINATION

There are four major organs of elimination: intestines, kidneys, skin and lungs. If these eliminating channels coordinate one with the other, the body drosses are thrown off in a normal way, and health is maintained. The liver and the lymphatic system, discussed in the next chapter, also play a major role in eliminating toxins from the body.

We can assist our lungs in the elimination process by practicing deep breathing, utilizing the diaphragm, that large dome-shaped muscle dividing the chest from the abdominal cavity. In diaphragmatic or abdominal breaths, the belly rises as we breathe in, contracts as we exhale; just the opposite of the way most of us have learned to breathe. As previously mentioned, acid waste is eliminated, in part, from the body in the form of carbon dioxide when we exhale. Deep breathing also moves lymphatic fluid, the carrier medium for our immune cells. Many of us are mouth breathers and need to relearn to inhale through the nostrils, whose tiny hairs filter out airborne particles, preventing them from reaching the lungs. Since the lungs are an organ of elimination designed to assist the body in riding itself of toxins, it is certainly advisable to refrain from adding to their toxic burden by not smoking. There are 47 different toxins in cigarette smoke, including the heavy metals nickel, cadmium, lead and arsenic. It has been established that "smoking causes more deaths in this country than AIDS, heroin, crack cocaine, alcohol, car accidents, fire and murder combined."[1]

We can assist our kidneys with their eliminative function by keeping them flushed through adequate intake of water. Adequate intake is generally 1/2 oz. per pound of body weight, although less may be required for the person whose diet consists predominantly of high water content foods (fruits and vegetables and their juices).

We eliminate toxins through the skin when we sweat. Any exercise that causes us to perspire is therefore helpful in this regard. Hydrotherapy, the use of saunas and the practice of massage also stimulate the skin, helping to open the pores and facilitate the elimination process.

The final organ of elimination is the intestines, through which solid wastes pass. Eating a diet high in fiber will facilitate elimination through this channel, for fiber, although it has no nutritional value, acts as sort of a whisk broom in the intestines, sweeping away debris which would otherwise accumulate, causing constipation. A high fiber diet is one that consists chiefly of fruits, vegetables and whole grains. Meat has no fiber. Diets consisting primarily of meat and processed, refined foods lack sufficient fiber to keep the colon free of accumulations. As fecal matter and mucus build up in the intestines, the bowel becomes underactive, and toxic wastes are then absorbed through the bowel wall into the blood stream. From there, they become deposited in the tissues, and thus the stage for degenerative disease is set.

Accumulations on the bowel wall also become a breeding ground for unhealthy bacteria. The normal balance of intestinal bacteria is 15-20% putrefactive (harmful, of which E. coli is a dominant strain) and 80-85% beneficial, of the Lactobacillus and Bifidobacterium varieties. Antibiotics destroy all bacteria, including the beneficial flora (bacteria) that synthesize B vitamins in the intestines. B vitamin deficiencies may therefore occur after administration of antibiotic therapy if valuable flora are not reimplanted in the intestines. Contrary to popular belief, this cannot be effectively accomplished by eating yogurt, as the dominant strain of lactobacillus in yogurt, bulgaricus, is of animal origin and not viable in the human intestines.

Random analysis of stool samples from apparently "healthy" people have shown a ratio of putrefactive to beneficial bacteria that is exactly the reverse of what it should be: 15-20% beneficial, 80-85% harmful. The proliferation of putrefactive bacteria can cause an overgrowth of the yeast germ Candida Albicans, which can give rise to any type and number of symptoms when present in the GI track of men or women. Also, absence of friendly bacteria in the intestines leads to impaired digestion, which in turn can lead to numerous other serious conditions created by the fermentation and putrefaction of undigested food. Undigested food particles in the blood are a significant factor in the development of allergies.

There are many reasons why most of us are short on friendly bacteria in the intestines. Among the most common are the use of antibiotics, mercury toxicity and the widespread consumption of refined carbohydrates and chlorinated water.

Incomplete elimination, along with imbalance of gut flora creates conditions in the body that are conducive to parasite infestation. Hulda Clark teaches us (in *Cure for All Cancers*) that the use of solvent-containing personal care products perpetuates such infestation. The presence of toxic metals (see chapter 6) in the body will make it very difficult to rid the body of parasites, fungi and other microorganisms.

Because accumulations on the bowel wall create toxic conditions in the body, it is felt advisable, especially for those on the SAD, to engage in some form of periodic colon cleansing — use of enemas, colonics or colemas (See Bernard Jensen's *Tissue Cleansing Through Bowel Management* for details on the colema board and the highly effective cleansing program in conjunction with which it is used). Enemas have limited effectiveness because they only cleanse the sigmoid area of the colon (see chart 3A).

Note also from the chart that areas of the colon correspond reflexively to areas of the body as a whole. Due to this reflexive relationship, a problem in one area of the body may he caused or perpetuated by an obstruction in the area of the colon reflexively related to it. The chart also shows the x-ray outlines of colons of people who *thought* they were in good health. As you can

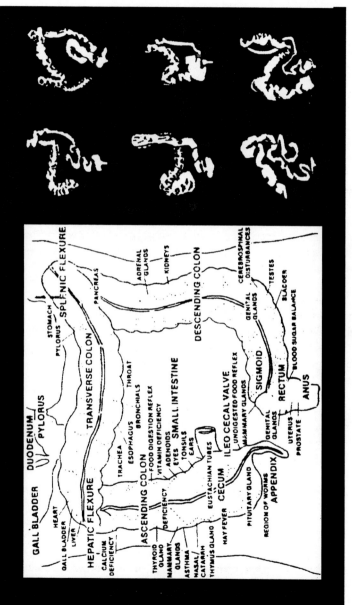

Chart 3A

see, each of these colons is distorted beyond recognition, and, although perhaps free of symptoms at the time of the photographs, their owners could hardly be considered "healthy." It has been said that health begins and ends in the colon.

If any of the eliminative channels — intestines, kidneys, lungs, lymph, liver or skin — is under-active, more wastes are retained in the body. And, as toxins accumulate in the tissues, increasing degrees of cell destruction take place.

Before leaving the subject of elimination, a word about the liver is in order. A major function of this organ is to filter toxins. The liver therefore may also be considered an organ of elimination, although it has many other functions as well. As long as its eliminative function is intact, the bloodstream remains pure. When the liver's ability to filter toxins becomes impaired, toxic substances enter the circulatory system and cause irritation (intestinal inflammation), destruction and eventual death. It has been said that man could live forever if his **liver** kept filtering. We shall look later at ways in which we damage our livers.

Dr. Alexis Carrel of the Rockefeller Institute theorized that the cell could live forever if kept free of its own waste. He designed and implemented a now classic experiment in which the heart tissue of a chicken was immersed in a nutrient solution that was changed daily. He kept the tissue alive for 29 years. At the time of its disposal, it was undamaged, youthful and healthy. The results of this experiment went a long way toward proving Dr. Carrel's hypothesis that if the body fluids are kept pure and proper elimination of cellular waste occurs, the cell will live indefinitely. The environment — or terrain — in which the cell lives seems therefore to have a huge amount to do with the health of that cell. Béchamp observed this more than a century ago.

VON LIEBIG/HENSEL

The Pasteur-Béchamp story is one I've told over and over in my classes. The suppression of Béchamp's research paved the way for the run-away growth of a giant medical-pharmaceutical monopoly, based on the false premise of monomorphic activity.

Just as important — and just as disillusioning — as the Pasteur/Béchamp story — is the Von Liebig/Hensel story which played out in Germany over a century ago. Von Liebig's work paved the way for the chemical trust to infiltrate and ultimately dominate the field of agriculture. To do that successfully, it was necessary to suppress Hensel's contrary findings. This story is told in the context of an article of mine that was published in 1995 in *Acres USA*. It also contains some interesting information on vitamin B12:

WHERE HAVE ALL THE MINERALS GONE?

In his fascinating treatise, "To B12 or Not to B12," David Yarrow asks the probing question, "Is this vanishing vitamin really a magnetic hormone?"

B12, isolated in 1948, is constructed from four basic life elements, carbon, oxygen, hydrogen and nitrogen, surrounding a cobalt atom. It is this mineral element which accounts for B12's magnetism. Cobalt is one of three naturally magnetic elements. The other two are nickel and iron.

B12 plays an important role in red blood cell formation. Yarrow suggests that the donut shape of the red blood cells is "highly suggestive of a magnetic function" since this shape is consistent with magnetic fields. He points out that the magnetic element, iron, forms the center of the hemoglobin molecule, just as cobalt forms the center of B12. He further suggests that the role of B12-cobalt is to "wind up the red cell magnetic field to activate iron's magnetic function." If such is the case, then iron cannot function properly in the absence of cobalt, for it will lack the requisite magnetic qualities to attract and bind oxygen. Oxygen, of course, is a basic necessity for life on this planet. Without it, cells cannot convert sugar to energy.

We can see then, how critical cobalt is to our very existence. And yet, the amount of the element needed for us to function optimally could fit on the head of a pin. The fact that Bl2 is needed only in minute amounts makes it more like a hormone than a vitamin. B12 is concentrated in the pineal gland of the body. This master endocrine gland sits atop the brain stem and is responsible for setting the time and rhythm of our hormonal ebb and flow. Secretions from the pineal gland are synchronized with the earth's resonant frequency, between 7 and 10 hertz or cycles per second. It is through the antenna of this gland that we are tied into the energy of the planet.

Providing the body with either too little or too much of the vital magnetic factor, cobalt, will result in an electrolyte imbalance that will adversely affect all basic body functions and ultimately lead to disease conditions. Electrolytes are mineral salts which are capable of conducting electricity when placed in solution. Electrolyte balance is crucial in maintaining the body's homeostatic mechanisms, which is a key factor in health maintenance. This balance, in turn, is dependent upon the presence of trace minerals such as cobalt in the environment.

We've been told that we get B12 only from animal sources. It's true that carnivores get B12 by eating herbivores. The B12 itself, however, is produced only by bacteria found in soil, water and in the gut of ruminant animals. (Herbivores culture the microbe in a special stomach called the "rumen"). B12 bacteria are highly sensitive to pH shifts and can survive only in an alkaline environment. This fact provides the key to the decline — and near disappearance — of B12 in our environment. The key is to be found in the increasing acidification of our soils. The use of chemical fertilizers and the effects of acid rain have caused a decrease in soil and water pH which has resulted in the die-off of bacteria necessary for the formation of B12. These soil bacteria or microorganisms are also necessary for the survival of all plant life, for they serve the vital function of breaking up and transmuting minerals for use by plants. When microorganisms disappear from the soil, so do minerals. Plants then starve. And ultimately so do we. Cobalt is one of the elements leached from our soils by acid rain and chemical fertilizers. According to Yarrow, both nickel and manganese can substitute for cobalt, forming false B12 analogues and increasing soil depletion of cobalt. Not only are cobalt and other trace minerals made unavailable to plants due to decreased pH, but toxic metals, such as aluminum and lead, are then taken up by plants in their place.

Yarrow's sobering conclusion is that B12 extinction is imminent, that its decline, along with that of trace minerals in our soils and geo-magnetism in the planet (a 50% drop in the earth's magnetic field in the last 500 years), represents a significant threat to our survival. His words are reminiscent of the repeated warnings issued to the governments of the earth since the late 1960s by John D. Hamaker (see his book, *The Survival of Civilization*). This brilliant engineer/ecologist had a profound grasp of the interrelationship between planetary ecology, the health of the individual and the rise and fall of civilizations. He understood the link between agricultural practices, physical and mental health, weather patterns and earth changes. And he, like Yarrow, saw the disappearance of soil microbes as the basic threat to our survival. The bottom line is that if we do not return the minerals to the soil, then Mother Nature will do it for us. She's done it before; in fact, does it in 100,000 year cycles and is, according to Hamaker, in the process of doing it again.

The way Mother Nature remineralizes the earth is by ushering in an Ice Age. When glaciers tumble over the terrain, they break up rocks, providing food for microorganisms, which, in turn, transmute minerals for use by plants. Over time, rock decays, producing highly mineralized soil. The Ice Age begins when soil minerals are depleted. It lasts 90,000 years and is followed by 10,000 years of civilization. Soil erosion takes place gradually over this 10,000 year period, as natural forces, such as wind and rain, deplete the soil of minerals. Modern man has stepped up the time table, it would seem, through his depletion and poisoning of the soils and grand-scale pollution of the atmosphere, so that we are now at the end of a 10,000 year inter-glacial period and on the brink of global catastrophe.

Our only hope for survival, according to Hamaker, lies in mobilizing the resources of all countries of the earth in a cooperative effort to remineralize the planet through the widespread use of "rock dust." The discovery that ground up rock could remineralize the soil was made accidentally by a German, Dr. Julius Hensel, in the late 1800s. Hensel was apparently the last person, prior to Hamaker, to publicly advocate soil remineralization through the use of rock dust. This miller, turned soil scientist, had one day accidentally ground up some rocks with flour and disposed of the useless mixture in his garden. He later noted accelerated growth and improved quality in the plants. He went on to commercially produce "stone meal" and write up his findings in a book called *Bread From Stones.* Unfortunately, stone meal was forced off the market and *Bread From Stones* was suppressed and even removed from libraries.

The opposition to Hensel's work and attack on it was led by the chemical industry. They had a vested interest in suppressing the truths revealed by Hensel, for they had profited immensely from contrary findings made many years earlier by another German, Professor Justis Von Liebig.

In 1840, Von Liebig published *The Organic Chemistry of Agriculture,* wherein he claimed that certain elements, notably N, P and K (nitrogen, phosphorus and potassium), should be added back to the soil to compensate for deficiencies and that acids would make the minerals more available to the plants.

Over the next ten years, the chemical companies started turning a handsome profit from sales of NPK fertilizers, widely used by farmers virtually everywhere to this day. Ironically, Von Liebig himself later realized the error of his teachings and officially published a retraction in the *Encyclopedia Britanica,* wherein he stated that adding *some* minerals back to the soil was insufficient, that plants needed the full spectrum of mineral elements (which, of course, is supplied in rock dust). Unfortunately, Von Liebig's revised findings were also suppressed, and they were omitted from subsequent editions of the *Encyclopedia Britanica.* Consequently, nutritionally incomplete acid chemical fertilizers, harmful to soil, continued to dominate in agricultural teaching and practice.

Today, altered soil pH, resulting from chemical fertilizers and acid rain, has hastened the demineralization of our soils and death of soil microorganisms. Two hundred years ago, our topsoil (the nutrient-rich ground cover) measured over three feet in depth. Today, we have less than six inches. The net result is sterile soil and malnourishment of all animals (and man) feeding off the products of the soil. Disease develops when enzyme systems are malfunctioning for lack of the mineral elements required to make enzymes. Among those minerals disappearing from the soil are the trace elements (such as cobalt) critical for electrolyte formation. The result is widespread electrolyte depletion, breakdown of homeostatic mechanisms and escalation of the degenerative disease process.

Mental, as well as physical, health is adversely affected, for mineral deficiencies and the subsequent breakdown of enzyme systems result in depletion of brain chemicals that leads to behavioral abnormalities. As minerals and soil microorganisms disappear, plants become sick and die, releasing CO_2 into the atmosphere. Dead forests burn easily. Forest fires result in oxidation of large quantities of atmospheric nitrogen, a major component of acid rain. The resulting "greenhouse effect" increases global warming — initially. What Hamaker taught us is that, in the long run, large scale evaporation of waters from tropical oceans will result in massive cloud coverage, blocking the warmth of the sun and increasing precipitation, and ultimately glaciation. According to Hamaker, "It's too late for soil "conservation:"

> *The money spent on conservation has been wasted because no one can conserve the soil and water but the microorganisms... The only answer is to make sure that the soil contains an abundance of available elements from the total natural mixture, and let the microorganisms pick and choose what they want, so that the natural balance of nutrients comes up through the plant life to us.(1)*

Hamaker's message fell on the deaf ears of world governments, but some among their peoples have heard his message and taken action. For more information on what is being done, what needs to be done and how to avert glaciation, I would recommend subscribing to *Remineralize the Earth*, a magazine that is published three times yearly (413-586-4429, www.remineralize-the-earth.org).

On a personal level, to compensate for the lack of minerals in our soils (and consequently in our foods), supplementation is recommended. Be aware, however, that many supplements can perpetuate or increase, rather than correct, imbalance by providing too much of certain elements, especially toxic ones. Also, minerals are often provided in forms that are not well utilized by the body. Therefore, I recommend emphasizing organic whole food supplements.

From the specific question of B12 scarcity to threat of global catastrophe, soil microorganisms are the common denominator. In the words of David Yarrow, "It's a grand irony that human survival may depend on a lowly microbe."

It's interesting to note that both Von Liebig and Pasteur confessed the error of their ways in the latter part of their lives. Von Liebig came to believe the soils need to have replacement of ALL, not just some of the minerals, but his efforts to set the record straight were foiled by the chemical trust that was profiting handsomely from his original findings that promoted N-P-K replacement. This fact is not well known, nor is Pasteur's death-bed confession about the terrain being more important than microbes. The "truth" that has been widely publicized and has been handed down to us is that which maintains the status quo in agriculture and medicine — and allows chemicals to dominate both fields.

From this information, we can see the huge contribution that high-yield chemical agriculture has made to the declining health of our planet by increasing toxicity and decreasing nutrient content of our food supply. Consumption of toxic, nutrient-depleted food has a decidedly adverse effect upon the internal terrain.

pH

No discussion of terrain would be complete without at least a brief explanation of pH (Potential of Hydrogen ion concentration). It is used to measure the relative acidity or alkalinity of substances by this scale:

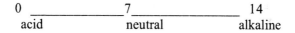

0	7	14
acid	neutral	alkaline

As the line indicates, a substance is neutral at 7. Distilled water has a pH of 7. The lower the pH, the more acid the substance.

The pH of our blood is neutral to slightly alkaline. According to the late Prof. Louis C. Vincent, pioneer in bioelectronics, the ideal blood pH lies between 7.0 and 7.2, though medical text books place it at 7.35 to 7.45. Any significant deviation from this range is fatal. The organism therefore will go to great lengths to protect the pH of the blood. If it starts to become too acid (as is so often the case with the SAD), then the body buffers it by adding some alkaline minerals — sodium, calcium, potassium, magnesium. If these minerals are not supplied in the diet in a usable form, they must be taken from the body's storehouses, its own tissues.

The primary alkaline mineral is sodium, which is stored in the liver. When the liver is depleted of sodium, it can no longer neutralize toxic acids, and, at this point, toxins get into the bloodstream. The endocrine glands take over (primarily the pituitary, thyroid and adrenals), and it becomes their task to direct the toxins to other eliminative organs — the lungs, skin, kidneys. In their efforts to take on this added chore, the glands go first into hyperfunction (over-activity) and then into hypofunction. In their hyperfunctioning stage, they enlarge and cause acute disease. In *Food Is Your Best Medicine,* Henry Bieler, M.D., points out that the enlarged pituitary can lead to migraines, blindness and epilepsy. Hyperthyroidism can give rise to skin and lung diseases, as well as growth disorders, and the hyperfunction of the adrenal glands can cause diarrhea and kidney troubles. *Hypo* function of these organs causes more health problems; those of a chronic nature.

When the liver has been depleted of 70% of its sodium (to provide alkaline substance to protect the pH of the blood), then the body stops pulling the mineral from it and goes to the muscles. When the muscles become depleted of sodium, they become flabby. At that point, the body begins to draw on its storehouse of calcium. Tissues, muscles and bones are robbed, giving rise to such degenerative diseases as arthritis, emphysema, osteoporosis and cancer.

The minerals needed by the body are in organic form. When I speak of sodium, I do not mean table salt — that is inorganic sodium chloride. Much of the food consumed in the SAD is mineral-poor, and many of the minerals that are ingested are inorganic and therefore not usable by the body.

When we eat a poor diet and subject the body to other stresses, we upset the critical pH balance. Such stress causes a reduction in hydrogen ion concentration in the tissues of the body. As the amount of hydrogen decreases, pH increases, creating an alkaline condition in the tissues. Hydrogen ions are then shifted to the blood, lowering its pH. It is at this point that the body is forced to draw from its own storehouses of alkaline mineral to protect the critical pH of the blood. Vincent has demonstrated that deviations from the ideal pH in blood, urine and saliva, along with deviations of other parameters (including oxidation/reduction), create different disease patterns. His work formed the basis of today's Biological Terrain Assessment (BTA), an effective assessment tool used by many alternative physicians.

Many diseases begin when tissue becomes too alkaline, causing a shift in pH in the blood. Alkalinity in an organ or tissue causes harmless microorganisms to reverse their polarity and become toxic, giving rise to such conditions as cancer. Different body tissues have different pH values. Cells with high metabolic activity normally tend to be acidic due to increased carbon dioxide production, while cells with a lower metabolic rate tend to be more alkaline. A cellular environment that preserves the slight alkalinity of the blood and slight acidity of most of the body tissues appears to be one that is health-promoting. The diet recommended to maintain or create this desired pH balance is one that is approximately 20% acid-forming and 80% alkaline-forming.

Basically, alkaline-forming foods are all vegetables (except legumes) and most fruits. The acid-forming foods include sugars, most grains, all meat and fish and most nuts.

Some foods are categorized differently by different authorities. It is generally agreed that millet is the only grain which is not acid-forming, though one authority (Herman Aihara, *Acid and Alkaline*) also lists buckwheat as alkaline-forming. Freshly picked corn is alkaline-forming, but generally corn is listed as acid-forming, for it becomes so within a short time after being picked. The consensus seems to be that sugars are acid-forming (though molasses and honey are considered by some to be alkaline-forming), vegetable oils alkaline-forming and nut oils acid-forming. There is widespread disagreement on dairy products: I have seen some charts list them as acid-forming, some list them as alkaline-forming and another as neutral. As previously stated, I believe the degree of acidity of these products depends upon the extent to which they have been processed, and I would therefore list commercial dairy products as acid-forming and raw ones as alkaline-forming.

While nuts are generally acid-forming, most authorities seem to agree that Brazil nuts and almonds are exceptions. Another area of disagreement about categorization of pH of foods is in regard to fruits: While all seem to agree that most fruits are alkaline-forming and that cranberries are one exception, plums, prunes and rhubarb are also listed by one source as further exceptions (Dr. Harold Reilly, *The Edgar Cayce Handbook for Health Through Drugless Therapy*). I cannot reconcile these discrepancies, except to state that differences in pH measurements can be the result of use of different measurement techniques. It is perhaps best to focus on the areas of agreement, drawing your own conclusions regarding the exceptions. Also, what is acid-forming for one person might not be for another, given differences in metabolism.

As regards the plum, while some authorities list it as acid-forming, the Japanese umeboshi plum (used widely in macrobiotics) has an alkalizing effect upon the system. Any fruit when cooked becomes acid-forming.

Eggs are generally listed as acid-forming. Most grains are acid-forming, while seeds (pumpkin, sunflower and sesame) are not. Sprouting both grains and seeds makes them more alkaline (and more digestible).

To summarize the categorization of foods according to pH, refer to the lists below. The items with the asterisks are those upon which there is not total agreement:

Alkaline-Forming
fruits (except cranberries, plums,* prunes,* rhubarb*)
all vegetables except legumes (and most dried peas and beans)
Brazil nuts, coconuts and almonds*
millet, buckwheat*
lima beans, soybeans
sprouted grains and seeds
honey

Acid-Forming
grains (except millet and buckwheat* and corn*)
all poultry, fish, meats and eggs
sugars and syrups (except honey)
nuts (except Brazils and almonds)
legumes and beans (except limas and soybeans)

There are good wholesome foods in both lists. What we need to aspire toward is selecting more foods (approximately 4/5 of our diet) from the top list. The ideal diet would maintain the gentle alkalinity of the blood and yield a 6.5 saliva value and a 6.8 urine pH, according to Vincent's research. Most degenerative diseases, he established, are the product of high (alkaline) blood and saliva pH and low (acid) urine pH, resulting largely from poor diet.

To get an idea of your body's pH, use special pH paper (which turns a different color for each number — the more alkaline, the darker) to check your urine and saliva first thing in the morning. Check the saliva upon awakening, before rising, and test the first urine of the morning. You will find that the urine pH will change rapidly and vary from day to day, depending upon what you recently ate. During a fast or cleansing diet, it will become temporarily quite acid as acid toxins are dislodged from tissue and carried out of the body. The pH of your saliva will take more time (probably many months) to change, for it more closely reflects what is happening at the cellular level.

It is not desirable to be too acid or too alkaline. Any imbalance stresses the system and ultimately leads to disease conditions. Please remember, when an organ is stressed, it first goes into hyperactivity and then into hypoactivity. Hyper function is associated with over-acidity, hypo function with over-alkalinity. In the hyper stage, we may well feel energetic, particularly if stimulants such as coffee, alcohol and cigarettes are used, but the net result is fatigue, resulting from decreased electrical energy to the organs. External stimulation is not a viable substitute for internal regulation. And for the body's regulatory functions to remain intact, we must know and follow the laws of the body, particularly as regards the cellular environment — the terrain — we create through the foods we eat and other lifestyle factors.

There are several factors that cause depletion of our alkaline reserve. Among them are:

- A high protein diet
- High levels of stress
- Highly processed foods

To build up our alkaline reserve, we want to:

- Eat plenty of fruits and vegetables
- Get fresh air and sunshine

When we exhale, we get rid of 300 times more acid than in any other way, so we want to be sure to exhale completely.

Think of pH as "Potential for Health." As we succeed in establishing a balanced pH in the body, we will be creating a cellular environment that is not conducive to the proliferation of microorganisms.

CHAPTER 4

Lympology

*"The body is primarily an electrical
or wave form system."*
Jack Tips

The organs of the immune system are generally referred to as lymphoid organs. They are concerned with the development, growth and deployment of white blood cells, the most important of which are the lymphocytes. The lymphocytes provide the body's line of defense against antigens. An antigen is any molecule the body identifies as "non-self" — virus, bacteria, fungus, parasite, pollen. Even a tissue transplant will be treated by the body as an antigen and rejected unless special measures are taken to bypass the rejection mechanism, usually by suppressing immune function.

The main bases of the immune system are the bone marrow, thymus, lymph nodes, liver and spleen. Auxiliary lymphoid organs are the tonsils, appendix and the Peyer's Patches found in the small intestines. So, the tonsils and appendix, which most of us have been taught have no purpose, and many of us have had removed, are actually part of our immune systems! Their purpose is to assist the body in elimination of catarrh, phlegm and mucous acid. The job of the Peyer's Patches is the collection of toxins.

The lymphatic system itself is the line of supply throughout the immune network. The system is linked up by lymph nodes. These are small structures shaped like beans and spread throughout the body, concentrated in the groin, abdomen, armpits and neck. The nodes serve as depositories for immune cells and as centers for disposing of the remains of dead microorganisms.

The lifeline for the lymphatic system is a network of vessels similar to, but separate from, blood vessels. These lymphatic vessels contain a clear fluid, lymph, which acts as a carrier for the immune cells. As illustration 4A shows, the lymphatic system looks rather like a tree, with the trunk running down the center front of the body, roots going down into the legs and branches extending into the head and arms. The lymphatic vessels form our "Tree of Life."

There are several types of white blood cells or leukocytes, including T cells, B cells and the "cell eaters" such as macrophages. Special immune cells associated with lymphoid tissue in the body are called lymphocytes. There are two types — T cells and B cells. Think of "T" as standing for "thymus." While all the lymphocytes originate in the bone marrow, helper T cells multiply and mature in the thymus gland. They act as stimulant cells, prompting other immune cells to action when the body's immune

The Lymphatic System

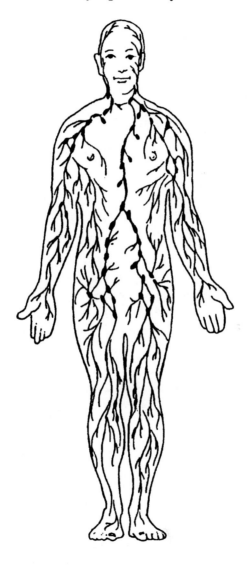

Illustration 4A

competence is compromised by the presence of antigens. These T cells are not themselves fighter cells. They serve more the function of commanding officer or general, mobilizing the troops to fight, then calling off the battle (suppressing the immune response) when danger is passed. Other types of T cells do actual hand-to-hand combat, attaching themselves to antigens. T cells called natural killer cells shoot out special proteins that punch holes in antigen walls, thereby killing them.

Think of "B" as standing for "bone marrow." The B cells originate in the bone marrow and mature either there or in immune organs other than the thymus. They are stationary fighter cells, and their primary role is the production of antibodies (specific chemical bullets) to fight bacterial invasion. An antibody is a unique kind of blood protein synthesized in lymphoid tissue in response to the presence of an antigen, which then circulates in the blood plasma. Remember this definition. It is highly pertinent to the discussion of blood proteins contained later in this chapter.

The phagocyte is a special type of cell that patrols the body, hunting down any type of antigen. Consider the phagocytic cells to be the "Special Forces" or "Green Berets" of the body's defense system. Macrophages are cells with phagocytic action that hide in the tissues. Monocytes are cells with phagocytic action that hide in the blood. Chart 4B shows the action of monocytes on antigens at the site of infection in the body. Note how these phagocytic cells act as killer scavengers, digesting the foreign antigens with PacMan-like action. After destroying an antigen, the macrophages present a piece of it to the T and B cells that study it and prepare weapons to be used against future invaders.

Most cells of the immune system use chemicals to attack invading organisms. When the invader is encountered, the B cells spawn a multitude of new cells known as plasma cells. Each one of these plasma cells is like a miniature chemical factory. They produce the antibodies that are released into the bloodstream. These antibodies will either knock out the antigen or coat its surface to tag it for identification by the phagocyte scavenger cells.

While all of this is going on, the helper T cells oversee the battle and, if necessary, call in reinforcements. Their function is a critical one, for the immune response would not be evoked without their activity. It is the T cells that are invaded by the AIDS virus. Suppression of the action of these key lymphocytes leaves

Lymphatic Activity

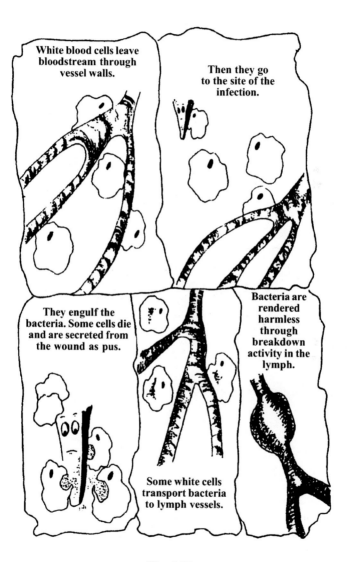

Chart 4B

the body open to all manner of infection, for the B cells will not launch an attack without the command of the T cells.

This cursory overview of immune function prepares us for a look at disease causation at the cellular level and a discussion of blood protein research.

BLOOD PROTEIN RESEARCH

Dr. C. Samuel West helps us to better understand the disease process. His own understanding began in 1974 when he learned from the second edition of Arthur C. Guyton's *Textbook of Medical Physiology* that blood proteins can produce the conditions at the cellular level that can cause death in just a few hours. Over the next six years, Dr. West developed a formula that explains life and death processes at the cellular level. The formula is introduced and the role of trapped plasma protein expounded upon in his informative book *The Golden Seven Plus One.* The remaining pages of this chapter explain West's theory and summarize his findings.

Before delving into Dr. West's blood protein research, it is important to know that everything in the body — all organs, all tissues, hard and soft – is composed of cells. When we fall ill or contract any type of disease or disorder, the cells die or become damaged.

Every cell in the body generates an electrical field. It is an actual electrical generator. We've known for a long time that the thought wave is electrical. It was demonstrated in the 1970s in a documentary film that amplified thought waves can influence the activity of matter. In this "train documentary," electrodes ran from a man's head to an electric train. It was found that the subject could control the movement of the train by thinking about it. His magnified thought waves could stop, start and speed up the electric train.

Kirlian photography allows us to view the electrical emanation radiating from all forms of matter. In inanimate objects, the radiation or "aura" is static, and in living beings, it is in constant motion. Changes in the aura result from changes in our thinking (an electrical phenomenon), among other things. And it has been found that signs of illness show up in the aura before they manifest as symptoms in the body. (More on Kirlian photography in chapter 12.)

Clearly the body is generating electrical current. Our strength and endurance depend upon the energy currents that run through our bodies. In order to keep the electrical generators in the body switched on, two conditions must be met:

1. The cells must have sufficient OXYGEN and GLU-COSE. Oxygen and glucose are major components in adenosine triphosphate (ATP) production. ATP is the fuel that keeps the generators going. It is the basic energy molecule of the cell.

2. The POTASSIUM inside the cell must remain high and SODIUM low.

Sodium outside the cell wall forces nourishment in. Potassium inside the cell forces waste out. It is the rotation of the minerals in and out of the cell that accounts for its electrical properties. This process of mineral rotation is set in motion by the sodium/potassium pump inside the cell. **The sodium-potassium pump is the electrical generator in the body.**

And, the ATP turns on the sodium-potassium pump. Without sufficient glucose and oxygen (components of ATP), the electrical generators (sodium-potassium pumps) are not turned on full force, and we therefore experience lack of energy. There is a literal short-circuit in the body. Now let's look at what is happening on a physical level to produce this condition, which is one of the first symptoms of disease.

Referring to the "Health/Disease" chart (4C), notice that section B represents the diseased state at the cellular level. The large white circles in the darkened area are cells. The darkened area itself represents an environment of excess fluid and excess sodium. This condition around the cells will cause them to drown from lack of oxygen (much as a plant dies when we water it excessively) and will upset the delicate sodium/potassium balance in and around the cells. Under these circumstances, the electrical generators cannot be kept going.

To have healthy cells, the body must be able (as shown in section A of the chart) to maintain a negative subatmospheric pressure condition or a "dry state" where there is no excess fluid, only enough to fill the crevices around the cells. The sub-atmospheric pressure condition is like a collapsed balloon. In this state, the cells remain close together, there is no bloating in the interstitial spaces (between the cells), and the cells stay in close contact with the capillary walls through which they receive oxygen and nutrients carried by the blood.

Referring once again to the chart, the black dots in the blood capillary represent blood proteins — albumins, globulins, fibrinogens — normal constituents of the blood plasma. These blood proteins continually seep through the tiny pores of the blood capillaries into the interstitial spaces. Since there is not enough pressure in these spaces to push the proteins back into the bloodstream, they must be continually removed through the lymphatic system. Note how the branches of the lymphatic capillary extend like fingers into the interstitial spaces.

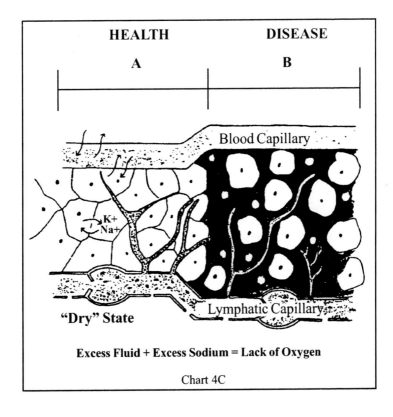

HEALTH   **DISEASE**

A   **B**

Blood Capillary

K+
Na+

"Dry" State

Lymphatic Capillary

Excess Fluid + Excess Sodium = Lack of Oxygen

Chart 4C

If the lymphatic system fails to operate properly, and the blood proteins get trapped in the interstitial spaces (as is the case in section B of our chart where the small white dots represent the proteins), the result is sickness or death. Death can occur very rapidly in the case of shock (as Guyton's medical text tells us): The blood capillaries dilate and dump the plasma proteins into the interstitial spaces all at once throughout the entire system. Since it is a rule that **body fluids follow blood proteins,** water leaves the bloodstream quickly, causing the collapse of the circulatory system. Death can occur within 24 hours. In the case of degenerative disease, the build-up of trapped plasma protein is less rapid and less generalized. The name of the disease will usually tell us the area of the body in which the blood proteins are trapped in the interstitial spaces.

Once the blood proteins enter the interstitial spaces, if they're not promptly carried off by the lymphatic capillaries, they will cause edema (water-logging) in the spaces between the cells. This happens because the proteins carry a negative charge and therefore attract the positive sodium ions from the bloodstream. Remember — **body fluids follow blood protein.** The main purpose of the blood proteins is to keep water in the bloodstream. However, when they get stuck in the interstitial spaces, the water remains there. And when this is the case, the white blood cells cannot ingest bacteria, and impaired immunity results. Remember the definition of antibody given earlier? — "a unique kind of *blood protein* that is synthesized in lymphoid tissue in response to the presence of an antigen and then circulates in the blood plasma." Since antibodies are proteins (of the globulin type), they are subject to getting stuck in the interstitial spaces like any other blood protein. When this happens, the body's immune response is suppressed, for its weapons (antibodies) are effectively unavailable, being "locked up" in the interstitial spaces.

The condition illustrated in section B of our chart, where we have excess fluid and excess sodium around the cells, upsets the sodium/potassium balance in and around the cells, causes a lack of oxygen and nutrients to the cells, and results in loss of energy, inflammation and pain. Excess sodium and lack of oxygen will reduce the electrical energy produced by the cells. Trapped plasma proteins upset the chemical balance of the body and literally cause a short circuit.

When the electrical generators of the body are switched on, we are healthy. HEALTH IS ENERGY. It is not merely an absence of symptoms. Many of us consider ourselves to be in good health and yet suffer from fatigue, which is one of the first signs of disease, for it is indicative of reduced electrical potential at the cellular level.

Sodium/potassium balance is critically important in maintaining health, for the sodium/potassium pump is the electrical generator of the body, and when it is switched off, the cells are deprived of oxygen, and ATP (fuel for the pump) production is impaired.

The late Dr. Max Gerson (whose Mexico clinic has successfully treated many terminal cancer patients through natural means for many years) also recognized the critical role of potassium in the body and taught that loss of potassium from the cells is the beginning of all degenerative disease. Gerson used the potassium in raw foods to correct the deficiency in the body and thus improve cellular respiration, which in turn mobilizes the white cells in their fight against antigens. A special potassium supplement is also used at the Gerson Clinic.

If trapped plasma protein causes disease, then it's logical to assume that we can prevent and possibly reverse the disease process if we know what causes the trapping and how to avoid it. Let's look then at the four basic causes of trapped plasma protein: poor nutrition, negative mental attitudes, inactivity and shallow breathing.

POOR NUTRITION

Dr. West tells us that trapped plasma protein is caused by foods that damage cells and make us thirsty. These foods include simple sugars, fats, animal products and alcohol. These act as poisons in the body, according to Dr. West. They cause the dilation of the blood capillaries, allowing the blood proteins into the interstitial spaces faster than the lymphatic system can remove them. The ideal diet, Dr. West tells us, consists primarily of fresh fruits and vegetables and sprouts. Fruits and vegetables are ideal food for five reasons: (1) They are alkaline-forming. (2) They are good sources of fiber. (3) They have a high water content. (4) They are an excellent source of glucose (needed for ATP production). (5) They are higher in vitamin and mineral content than any other food. A meatless diet is ideal for cleansing purposes, but not necessarily for maintenance (see chapter 9).

NEGATIVE MENTAL ATTITUDES

I have already mentioned the fact that shock can result in death within 24 hours by causing the blood capillaries to dilate and the plasma proteins to flood the interstitial spaces, bringing water from the bloodstream with them. On a smaller scale, stress has the same kind of effect upon the body. Negative thoughts act as mental poisons upon the body and cause trapped plasma protein. (More on this subject in chapter 12.)

PHYSICAL ACTIVITY

Just walking around provides enough stimulation to the lymphatic system to allow for some movement of plasma proteins out of the interstitial spaces. This minimal activity is enough to keep us alive. When we're at rest, the lymph system can drain 1-2 ml. of dead fluid per minute. During activity, it can drain 20 ml. We can therefore see why exercise is important. And there seems to be a special value to aerobic forms of exercise, for "unless we engage in some activity that causes us to breathe deeply, we will have trapped plasma protein, regardless of what else we do." A gentle bouncing motion, which can be comfortably maintained by doing a "soft walk" (alternating weight from the ball of one foot to the other) on a rebounder or mini-trampoline, is effective in promoting lymphatic circulation. The main function of the lymphatic system is to keep the blood proteins circulating. Exercise assists in this function. The bedridden patient can be benefited by the gentle bouncing motion created by having someone jump up and down on his bed. The wheelchair-bound person will reap the beneficial results of someone else jogging on the rebounder if he will place his feet on the jumping surface while the other is doing the exercise. Dr. West makes extensive use of the rebounder in his work and refers to it as a "lymphasizer."

SHALLOW BREATHING

The lungs serve as a sort of suction pump for the lymphatics. Deep breathing moves lymphatic fluid very effectively, and it floods the cells with oxygen, which enables them to convert glucose to ATP (needed to fuel the electrical generator, the sodium/potassium pump).

According to lymphologist Dr. Jack Shields, deep breathing drains lymph fluid ten to fifteen times more effectively than any other activity. Most of us do not breathe properly, as was previously discussed. The chest breather never fills his lower lungs, that portion that should be supplying 80% of the oxygen to our bodies. Our exhalations are likewise incomplete, which causes us to retain acid waste that otherwise would be expelled in the form of carbon dioxide. Re-birthers tell us that most of us are chronic hypoventilators, taking too little oxygen into our systems. This habit, they say, has its roots in the birth trauma when the doctor held us upside down and smacked our bottoms to shock the system into taking its first breath after the umbilicus had been abruptly severed moments before. Our first breath therefore was associated with trauma.

Because of its effect upon lymphatic flow, breath is the major controlling factor in our level of energy and our immune functioning. In a very real sense, oxygen is our most important nutrient. Try breathing in to the count of 5, holding to the count of 20 and exhaling to a 10 count. Your lymph will shoot through the vessels like a geyser. Do this ten times in a row, three times daily. It will nourish and protect the body. If it makes you dizzy, you need it — toxins are being stirred up and removed. Lack of oxygen at the cellular level is a major cause of pain and degenerative disease.

Breath is life. The old Indian, when he was ready to leave his body at the point of death, sat motionless under a tree and took in very shallow breaths to hasten his demise.

I have spoken of trapped plasma protein as a cause of degenerative disease. Before summarizing, I would like to say a few words about injuries: If we accidentally smash our thumb with a hammer, what is the first thing we do, that we instinctively do? We grab the thumb (and say ouch!). But not for long. Soon we let go, reasoning that we should wash it, put ice on it, a band-aid or whatever. And, as we're ministering to the injured finger, what is happening? It is swelling up. Why? Because damaged cells produce poison — histamine. A poison dilates the blood capillaries and lets the blood proteins in faster than the lymphatic vessels can carry them away. A more effective way to handle such an injury would be to continue holding onto the smashed finger. Hold it tightly for up to twenty minutes. Within twenty minutes, the poisons have stopped attacking the capillaries. After that, you can let go, do whatever you like, and expect to experience little to no pain and swelling.

If poor nutrition, negative mental attitudes, physical inactivity and shallow breathing cause trapped plasma protein, then it stands to reason that exercise, positive thinking, good nutrition and deep breathing will prevent it and help to reverse it. Sustained pressure (as described above) will also help dissipate trapped blood proteins, as will massage and light stroking motions. Electricity has also been found to break up clusters of trapped blood proteins. Clusters tend to form when the energy fields remain reduced in the spaces around the cells, and, once clusters have formed, the lymphatics have a hard time removing them. In *The Golden Seven Plus One,* Dr. West describes the work of Dr. Joseph Waltz, Director of the Department of Neurological Surgery at the St. Barnabas Hospital in New York. Dr. Waltz was able to help patients with cerebral palsy, multiple sclerosis and polio through electrical stimulation of the spinal cord. In this book, Dr. West gives us a system of lymphasizing (using the rebounder) designed to maximize lymphatic stimulation, dissipation of trapped plasma protein and pain reduction. He notes that the gentle, bouncing motion on the rebounder creates an electrical field that can be used to magnify thought waves (as was done in the train documentary previously mentioned) and accelerate healing. If the patient will think positive thoughts of healing and direct them at a specific body part, while simultaneously stroking that part and maintaining his "soft walk" and deep breathing on the rebounder, he can affect positive changes in the targeted body area. See Dr. West's book for details.

It should also be noted that trapped plasma protein can cause obesity. Dr. West states that some people seem to have a "loose cellular structure" and are therefore very prone to retaining extra water as a result of the blood protein clusters that form readily in their bodies. We can retain up to 21 gallons of excess fluid in the interstitial spaces — that's a lot of added weight. So, for the sake of your health and your appearance, be aware of the practices that cause trapped plasma protein, and consider adopting a more healthful lifestyle. There are many reasons to stimulate lymph flow and many ways to do it, as listed below:

WHY STIMULATE LYMPH FLOW?

1. IMPROVE IMMUNITY
2. IMPROVE CIRCULATION
3. DECREASE EDEMA/SWELLING
4. REDUCE MASSES (such as cysts and fibroids)
5. REDUCE CELLULITE
6. REDUCE TOXICITY
7. DECREASE PAIN
8. CALM THE NERVOUS SYSTEM
9. INCREASE ENERGY LEVELS
10. ACCELERATE HEALING OF INJURIES

TO STIMULATE LYMPH FLOW:

1. DRINK PLENTY OF PURE WATER AND FRESH JUICES
2. EXERCISE ON A REBOUNDER DAILY
3. DO BREATHING EXERCISES REGULARLY
4. ELIMINATE REFINED FOODS & DAIRY PRODUCTS
5. KEEP ACID-FORMING FOODS (meat, nuts, grains) TO A MINIMUM (no more than 20% of the diet)
6. USE APPROPRIATE HERBAL &/OR HOME-OPATHIC PREPARATIONS & SUPPLEMENTS
7. USE A SLANT BOARD DAILY (head lower than feet)

8. HAVE REGULAR COLONICS (colon cleansing)
9. EAT PLENTY OF FIBER (fruits, vegetables, whole grains) TO CLEANSE THE GI TRACT
10. CONSIDER ELECTRO-LYMPHATIC THERAPY WITH MANUAL DRAINAGE (such a device applies a negative electrical charge to the tissues to disassociate blood proteins and cellular debris. The "manual drainage" consists of special lymphatic massage)

CHAPTER 5

Immunizations

*"The greatest medicine of all
is to teach people not to need it."*
unknown

The word "immunization" is actually misleading, for to "immunize" is "to render immune" or resistant to disease. To vaccinate is to inoculate with a vaccine for the purpose of producing immunity against disease. To inoculate is "to introduce the virus of a disease or other antigenic material into the body in order to immunize, cure or experiment" *(The Concise American Heritage Dictionary)*. We often use the word "immunize" interchangeably with "vaccinate" or "inoculate," indicating our acceptance of the belief that vaccinations or inoculations confer immunity against disease upon the recipient. This commonly held belief may be unfounded and invalid, as will be illustrated in the remaining pages of this chapter. Therefore, the word "vaccinations" rather than "immunizations" will be used henceforth.

While there are no national vaccination laws in the U.S., there is a high degree of uniformity among the states on vaccination policy. All 50 states in the U.S. require vaccination against traditional childhood diseases as a prerequisite to public school admission. As of January, 1999, the Routine Immunization Schedule recommended by the Advisory Committee on Immunization Practice and the American Academy of Family Physicians included the following vaccinations for children from birth to 16 years of age:

DPT – diptheria, tetanus, pertussis
   or Dtap – diptheria, tetanus, acellular pertussis
Hib – Haemophilus influenza, type B
HBV – hepatitis B virus
MMR – measles, mumps, rubella
IPV – inactivated polio virus
TD – tetanus and diptheria
V – varicella (chicken pox)

MEASLES

The live measles vaccine was introduced in 1963. It is typically administered as part of the MMR (Measles, Mumps, Rubella) vaccine. By the time of its introduction, the measles mortality rate had already dropped significantly — from 13.3 in 100,000 in 1955 to 0.3 in 100,000. Historically, this disease, like similar ones, has resulted in relatively high rates of complications and deaths among adolescents and young adults, while doing no permanent or prolonged damage to the pre-adolescent youth. The downgrading of a disease such as measles from killer status to "routine childhood disease" is indicative of the development of "herd" immunity in youngsters where the disease, when contracted, follows a benign, self-limited course. Measles is typically characterized by a skin rash (pink spots) and high fever. More serious complications can include eye and ear inflammations, pneumonia, and, in rare cases, encephalitis. Pneumonia is the most common complication. In itself it, too, is benign and self-limiting. Dr. Richard Moskowitz, medical and homeopathic physician, tells us:

> Ironically, what the measles vaccine has done is to reverse the historical or evolutionary process to the extent that measles is once again a disease of adolescents and young adults, with a correspondingly higher incidence of pneumonia and other complications and a general tendency to be a more serious and disabling disease than it usually is in younger children.(1)

The measles vaccine is usually administered in a single dose after one year of age.

MUMPS

Mumps is a viral disease, usually self-limiting, requiring no medical treatment. Once a child has contracted mumps, he will usually not develop the condition again, for acquisition of the disease typically confers lifetime immunity on the recipient. Symptoms of mumps include fever, headache, loss of appetite and swelling of salivary glands. Because of the benign nature of the disease, 16 of our 50 states do not require that the mumps portion of the MMR be given. Where required, one dose after the first birthday is usually given.

As with measles, Dr. Moskowitz tells us that mumps is now affecting an increasing number of adolescents and young adults. The chief complication, occurring in 30-40% of post puberty males, is "acute epididymo-orchitis," which usually results in testicular atrophy on the affected side of the body. Also adversely affected are the pancreas and ovaries.(2)

RUBELLA (GERMAN MEASLES)

The symptoms of rubella (three day rash, fever, sore throat, mild "cold") are at times so mild in young children as to go undiagnosed. In older children and in adults, however, the disease can produce more severe symptoms, including arthritis and joint pain. The vaccine itself has also been known to cause such symptoms. The greatest risk posed by rubella is in exposure of a pregnant woman, for if she contracts the disease in her first trimester of pregnancy, damage to the developing embryo in the form of Congenital Rubella Syndrome (CRS) can result. The rubella outbreak of 1964 resulted in a relatively high incidence of CRS, with an estimated 20,000 babies being affected. A mass "immunization" program followed in 1969. Rubella vaccine, like the measles vaccine, was once administered in a single dose after 12 months of age. Since January, 1999, however, a second shot between 4 and 6 years of age has been recommended.

Like measles and mumps, rubella is a relatively benign, self-limited disease of early childhood that poses little to no threat to young children. The MMR vaccination, however, has transformed these diseases into more serious ones that are now affecting the very age groups (adolescent and young adult) most in need of protection from them. There is strong evidence of a link between the MMR vaccination and autism, despite government claims to the contrary.

DIPHTHERIA

Unlike measles, mumps and rubella, diphtheria and tetanus are serious diseases that can be fatal. Diphtheria vaccination is typically administered as part of the DPT inoculation (Diphtheria, Pertussis, tetanus) or the newer DTaP. Diphtheria and tetanus vaccines are not made from the living disease germs themselves but rather from toxic substances associated with them. Tetanus and diphtheria "toxoids" therefore seek to vaccinate not against the diseases themselves but rather against the systemic effect of the original poisons. Both of these vaccines have been in use for a long time with a low incidence of reported problems stemming from their effects.

The necessity of the diphtheria vaccine is questionable, however, when we consider that the disease has nearly disappeared from this continent. The mortality rate had, in fact, *dropped by 50% prior to development of a vaccine* against diphtheria. And yet, today, all 50 states require 3-5 doses, the last one usually given after the fourth birthday. Tetanus was likewise disappearing prior to the introduction of the vaccine. Both diseases, furthermore, are easily controlled by application of appropriate sanitation measures.

Evidence shows that the child who has not been vaccinated against diphtheria is no more susceptible to the disease than his "fully immunized" counterpart. The Chicago Board of Health reported that in a 1969 outbreak of diphtheria, 25% of the children who contracted the disease had received all of the required vaccinations, and another 12% had been given one or more doses of the vaccine, enough to show "serological evidence of full immunity." Another 18% had been partially vaccinated, making a total of 55% affected children who had been totally or partially "immunized" and yet developed the disease.(3)

TETANUS

Tetanus is technically not a childhood disease. It is a bacterial infection that can produce muscle spasms (spasms in the jaw = "lockjaw") and neurological symptoms. The worldwide mortality rate is 30-50%, with the disease being particularly prevalent in tropical countries. Forty-seven states require 1-5 inoculations of the tetanus virus, starting at age 2 months.

The tetanus vaccine may interfere with the immune response and has been linked with peripheral neuropathy, allergic reactions and laryngeal paralysis.

PERTUSSIS

Pertussis, also known as whooping cough, is considered the most virulent of the childhood diseases. The predominant symptom of this potentially life threatening disease is a paroxysmal cough. A fever is also present. Frequency and severity of the disease had begun to decline significantly before the widespread use of the killed virus vaccine in 1957. In 1943, in fact, C.C. Dauer, epidemiologist, had remarked that if the mortality rate from pertussis were to decline at the then prevailing rate during the next 15 years, it would be "extremely difficult" to statistically correlate its decline with use of the vaccine (developed in 1936). Today, however, 39 states require 3-5 doses of the injectible vaccine beginning at 2 months of age.

Pertussis has become the most controversial of the vaccinations due to claimed adverse effects, which include central nervous system damage and hematological disturbances. The vaccine, while posing high risk, offers questionable immunity: According to the Center for Disease Control, of 759 cases of pertussis reported in infants in 1988, 49% *had been fully immunized.*

POLIOMYELITIS

Ninety percent of persons infected with the poliomyelitis virus exhibit *no symptoms* and only 1-2% of the children infected exhibit "classic" symptoms of the disease, meaning paralysis. Even at the zenith of the polio epidemic in this country in the 1950s, 2/3 of the reported cases of polio were of the non-paralytic type, characterized by excess mucus, headaches, fever and "aches and pains that come and go." Polio vaccination is now required nationwide in 3-4 doses. It once came in two forms: a killed virus injection developed by Dr. Jonas Salk in 1955 and an orally administered live virus developed by Dr. Carl Sabin in 1960. The oral vaccine is no longer being produced for use in the U.S.

Aggressive vaccination programs are usually credited with virtually wiping out polio, with statistics reflecting a dramatic drop in the disease. In 1952, there were 57,879 reported cases and only 19 in 1971. That looks, at first glance, like a giant success attributable to the vaccines. Let's take a closer look:

When polio was in its heyday and running rampant, diagnosis of the disease could be made if the above listed non-paralytic symptoms persisted for a period of only *24 hours.* Look again at these symptoms: muscle aches, excess mucus, headaches and fever. Since there are 66 other diseases that produce the same symptoms, and there was no test upon which to make a definitive, differential diagnosis, it is reasonable to believe that numerous people might have been diagnosed as having polio who may only have had a cold or some such benign ailment.

One huge factor in the rapid decline in the incidence of reported polio cases has been a change in the required duration of symptoms for a condition to qualify as being diagnosed as polio. At the start of the 1960s (when the Sabin vaccine was introduced), to be classified as "polio," the above cold-like symptoms had to persist for *30 days* rather than 24 hours! As one can imagine, this resulted in a drastic drop in the number of reported cases. Also, in 1961, the incidence of a new disease, "aseptic meningitis" rose in direct proportion to the decline in polio cases. It is interesting that the symptoms of aseptic meningitis are *exactly the same as the symptoms of polio* and, we are told that both diseases are said to come from the same virus.(4) In fact, the same source cites statistics from a 1961-62 California medical journal that reports zero polio cases, with a footnote stating, "All such cases now reported as *aseptic menin-gitis!*"(5)   So, was it the vaccine or the re-defining of the criteria for diagnosing polio that accounted for the "conquest" of the disease?

Dr. Moskowitz points out that a herd immunity had already begun to develop against polio prior to the introduction of the vaccine and that "immunity ... was already as close to being universal as it can ever be."(6)   Although Dr. Moskowitz states that the polio vaccine is "about as safe as any vaccine can be,"(7) Dr. Salk himself (who ironically became paralyzed) testified in front of Congress in 1980 that *95% of all polio cases* in the preceding 10 years had been *caused by the vaccine!*

The polio vaccine and all of the others discussed in this chapter, plus hepatitis B (HeP) and Haemophilus influenza type B (Hib) are now recommended for preschool children. In fact, "the American Academy of Pediatrics now recommends **21** vaccinations for children by the time they're in the first grade."(8) The HeP vaccine, first administered between birth and two months of age, has been linked to immunological and neurological disorders. Hib is purported to reduce the incidence of meningitis. However, much evidence to the contrary can be accessed on the Internet. One site (http://www.pslgroup.com/dg/fc486.htm) gives details on a report from the *British Medical Journal* linking the haemophilus meningitis vaccine to the development of insulin dependent diabetes.

A NEW POLIO

In the August 1996 edition his newsletter *Second Opinion,* William Campbell Douglass, M.D., presented evidence that the disorder we call Chronic Fatigue Syndrome is really a form of polio. Here's the reasoning behind this theory:

The polio virus, once ingested, reproduces in the small intestine. The use of vaccines, especially the oral Sabin vaccine, causes the original polio virus to be displaced by a related one called Coxsackie. Coxsackie viruses have been isolated from CFS patients, giving birth to a new type of non-paralytic polio.

Dr. Douglass points out that before the Salk and Sabin vaccines, there were only 3 polio viruses. Now, due to the disruption of the intestinal terrain caused by these vaccines, there are no less than 72 strains that can give rise to polio-like diseases. Rather than having been eliminated, then, polio has *changed.* It stands to reason that when we change the terrain (with vaccines), we change the form of microorganisms and thereby create new diseases.

The "new polio" gained momentum after the introduction of the vaccines and has been recognized by neurologists for 40 years, according to Douglass, who states flatly, "We now know that CFS is not a new disease, but simply an 'aborted form' of the more serious paralytic polio. There's no doubt about it." He goes on to say that the neurological nature of CFS can be demonstrated by the presence of lesions in the brain as revealed by MRI, and that other neurological diseases — MS, ALS, Tourette Syndrome, Guillain Barre Syndrome, learning disabilities, idiopathic epilepsy, etc.— may well be forms of polio brought on by the vaccines.

HOW VACCINATIONS WORK

According to the 1986 *Red Book,* the pediatrician's reference book on the subject, "The goal [of vaccinations] is to mimic the natural infection by evoking an immunologic response that presents little or no risk to the recipient."(9)   Many authorities seriously question both the effectiveness and the safety of the practice of vaccinating against disease. Objections are based, in part, on the arguments already mentioned — that disease rates were declining prior to the introduction of vaccines and the fact that many of the childhood diseases against which we routinely vaccinate are innocuous and self-limiting and therefore should be allowed to run their course. There is also the disturbing fact that many diseases have continued to appear in highly "immunized" populations. Dr. Moskowitz postulates that vaccines offer only partial or temporary immunity, but observes that there is no way to tell how long such immunity will last. In addition to "mimicking the natural infection," vaccines also produce their own sets of symptoms which, many experts tell us, may be more serious than the original disease.

Dr. Robert Mendelsohn, M.D., practicing pediatrician for 25 years, as well as others in the field of holistic medicine, including Moskowitz, have expressed the opinion that vaccinations may have the long-term effect of damaging the immune system. According to Mendelsohn, "The only proven characteristic of vaccines is their devastating adverse effects."[10] Far from enhancing immunity, it is argued by Moskowitz, vaccinations may serve only to drive the disease deeper into the tissues, creating a *chronic* condition, wherein our response to the disease actually becomes progressively weaker. Vaccines typically involve the injection of viruses *directly into the bloodstream,* whereas in the normal course of the disease process, these organisms find their way into the body through one of its orifices. Such ports-of-entry are equipped with *filters* to protect the bloodstream. By injecting the virus directly into the blood, we "give it free and immediate access to the major immune organs, without any obvious way of getting rid of it ... [and thus] we have accomplished what the entire immune system seems to have evolved in order to prevent."[11] The result is *immune SUPPRESSION,* the opposite of the claimed effect of the vaccination. Vaccinations result in the injected virus becoming permanently incorporated into the genetic material of the cell. Any antibodies produced by the body to combat that virus will therefore be directed against its own cells, resulting in autoimmune disease. Dr. Moskowitz concludes his argument by stating:

> If what I am saying turns out to be true, then what we have done by artificial immunizations is essentially to trade off our acute, epidemic diseases of the past century for the weaker and far less curable chronic diseases of the present, with their amortizable suffering and disability.[12]

Often the association between the vaccination and the symptoms created by it is not made due to the time lapse between inoculation and the onset of symptoms, the parents' lack of information regarding the connection, and the doctor's hesitancy in suggesting a causative link. Dr. Moskowitz suggests that homeopathy can be a valuable tool for *diagnosis,* as well as treatment of vaccine-related disorders. He gives some brief case histories, describing how symptoms subsided rapidly after administration of a single dose of the appropriate homeopathic dilution of the virus.

BUBBLE, BUBBLE, TOIL AND TROUBLE

As of 1988, there were 19 licensed vaccines in this country, including the 7 already described. There are many more today. These vaccines contain either a live or killed infectious agent, usually a virus or bacteria, as well as sterile water (used as a suspending agent), preservatives (including formaldehyde and mercury derivatives), stabilizers, antibiotics and adjuvants (aluminum phosphate). Hannah Allen tells us that the materials from which the "vaccines, serums and biologicals" are produced include:

1. rotten horse blood (for diphtheria toxin and antitoxin)
2. macerated cancerous breasts
3. sweepings from vacuum cleaners (for asthma and hay fever)
4. pus from sores of diseased animals
5. metallic poisons
6. powdered insects
7. mucous from the throats of children with colds and whooping cough
8. decomposed fecal matter from typhoid patients
9. sewage
10. urine
11. fecal matter
12. garbage
13. dishwater[13]

Is it really scientific or even rational to believe that having the above items injected into our bloodstream will confer immunity from disease?? It may not be rational, but it is big business in this country and worldwide, and we might therefore suspect vested interest rather than disease prevention as a prime motivating factor in promotion of vaccinations.

It is not surprising, in view of the above list, to note that vaccinations have actually been linked with development of such virulent diseases as Epstein-Barr Virus (EBV) and AIDS. As reported by Richard Leviton, the time-table looks something like this:

1985:   A scientist at Harvard's School of Public Health revealed that an AIDS-type virus (STLV-3) had been found in the African green monkey whose kidney cells were used to culture oral polio virus.

1987:   The London times reported that the prevalence of smallpox vaccinations over 13 years in 7 African nations triggered the AIDS virus outbreak there.

1988:   The *British Medical Journal* in a study of 200 patients with chronic EBV [Epstein-Barr virus], reported that it was caused by the live rubella virus found in the vaccine.(14)

THE HISTORICAL PERSPECTIVE

Preventive vaccination was first promoted in 1796 by Dr. Edward Jenner of England who developed a cowpox vaccination against smallpox. Use of his vaccine lead to massive outbreaks of the disease, and it was therefore banned by 1837.

Vaccinations are no longer compulsory in England, Germany or Sweden, and it's reported that since the decline in pertussis immunizations, hospitalizations and death rates from the disease have fallen in England.

Vaccinations were made non-compulsory in England due largely to the findings of Professor Alfred Russel Wallace, Anthony Robbins tells us.(15)   Dr. Wallace was asked by *Encyclopedia Brittanica* to write an article about how smallpox was wiped out by vaccinations. In his investigations, Robbins tells us, Dr. Wallace found that in countries where the vaccine was introduced, smallpox multiplied *15 times and that 65-70% of the people who contracted the disease had been vaccinated against it.* He wrote up these findings in a chapter called "The Pursuit of Evil," part of a larger volume entitled *The Wonderful Century.* The interesting thing, Robbins states, is that this chapter just happens to have been eliminated from all copies of this book found in the U.S., except one: The one complete volume is housed at Yale University. It may not be checked out, but can be read only on the premises in a locked room. Do you get the impression that information is being withheld on the subject?? As regards smallpox, it is also an interesting, little-known fact that Dr. Charles A.R. Campbell, who was recommended for the Nobel Prize around the turn of the century, discovered that the disease was caused by the bite of a blood-sucking insect, the bedbug, that it was not infectious nor contagious and that vaccinations do not prevent it.

THE LEGAL PERSPECTIVE

Prior to 1988, there was no nationwide mandated reporting system requiring reports to be filed on adverse reactions to vaccinations. Therefore, we have no accurate data on the subject. As things stand now, it is unknown how many of the 67,000 infants vaccinated weekly in the U.S. may be suffering from adverse reactions. Barbara Fisher, co-author of *DPT: A Shot in the Dark* and mother of a DPT vaccine injured child, founded D.P.T. (Dissatisfied Parents Together) in 1982 for the purpose of enhancing public awareness and initiating legislative action. In their book, she and co-author Harris Coulter estimate as many as 943 deaths and 11,666 cases of long-term damage from DPT vaccinations.

In his book *Dangers of Compulsory Immunizations: How to Avoid them Legally,* attorney Tom Finn cites the legal aspects, precedents and strategies of avoidance of vaccinations. He tells us that the courts have proclaimed that consumers must be adequately warned of the dangers of vaccines by the drug manufacturers, and that failure to give such warning opens them up to liability for injuries. He adds an interesting perspective on that ruling:

> It seems inconsistent to require the manufacturer to warn the consumer of the potential dangers connected with the vaccine's use and then compel an individual to be injected against their will. If the consumer is not allowed to make this choice because of a compulsory immunization statute, then the government is exposing itself to liability for any resulting injuries either under the theory that they're forcing the inoculation on the party or under the theory that the government has warranted that the drug is safe. It could be argued that the government has given its seal of approval to the vaccination by compelling individuals under penalty of law to be vaccinated.(16)

While all states require vaccinations as a prerequisite to public school admission, exemptions may be granted for medical reasons in all 50 states. Religious exemptions are allowed in all states except West Virginia and Mississippi, and philosophical exemptions may now be granted in 22 states. These exemptions offer a way out for parents choosing not to expose their children to the potential dangers of compulsory vaccinations.

The three major manufacturers of vaccines — American Cyanamide, Lederle and Wyeth — have had hundreds of lawsuits filed against them since 1984. Many have been settled out of court, with a ban on publicity. Of those that have gone to court, the majority of rulings have been in favor of the manufacturers. In 1987, the U.S. Department of Justice intervened as a 'friend of the court' in support of Wyeth Laboratory, thus overturning a $2.1 million damage decision that had been rendered in favor of a DPT-injured child. Several large monetary settlements have been awarded to injured parties, including $15 million (Graham vs. Wyeth, 1987) to a child who became retarded after his first DPT shot.

In 1986, the U.S. Congress set up a national no-fault vaccine injury compensation fund. Although doctors in this country are legally required to report suspected cases of vaccine damage to the Vaccine Adverse Event Reporting System (VAERS), the vast majority (90%, according to the FDA) do not, as they fail to recognize the connection between a patient's physical complaints and the vaccination(s) he or she received. None-the-less, 12,000 to 14,000 vaccine reactions (including hundreds of deaths) *are* reported each year to VAERS. The *actual* number of vaccine-related adverse reactions may therefore well be as high as 140,000 a year. As of 2002, VAERS has paid out over $1 billion in compensation, with thousands of cases yet to be resolved.

Medical historian Harris Coulter, Ph.D., claims that vaccines cause encephalitis (inflammation of brain tissue). When nerves that control breathing become damaged in an infant, crib death can occur, If damage is less severe, the child may develop asthma. Asthma has been found to be 6 times more prevalent in children receiving the pertussis vaccine than in those not receiving it. "When childhood vaccination rates in Australia dropped by 50% after vaccination was made non-mandatory, SIDS [crib death] cases also dropped by 50%. In 1975, Japan moved the age of first vaccination up to two years (two months is the norm for first vaccination in the U.S.), and since then, crib death and infantile convulsions have virtually disappeared."(17)

More information on the dangers associated with vaccinations is available through the Vaccine Research Institute, P.O. Box 4182, Northbrook, Illinois 60065. They publish a list of reference articles available for $3.00.

The theory that vaccinations can confer immunity against disease is an outgrowth of the theory that germs cause disease which was explored in chapter one. If, as suggested, autotoxemia is, instead, the root cause of disease because it creates a cellular environment conducive to the proliferation of germs, then the entire theoretical framework supporting vaccinations (and the whole of the medical model) proves unsound. And, it can be readily seen how the vaccines add to the body's toxic burden, thus *reducing immunity* rather than enhancing it.

There is growing evidence of the problems associated with vaccinations. At the end of 1990 Medline, the National Library of Medicine database, had 1,778 citations on the adverse effects of vaccinations. At the end of 1999 it had 3,816 such citations. According to Viera Scheibner, author of *Vaccination: The Medical Assault on the Immune System,* "Immunizations, including those practiced on babies, not only did not prevent any infectious diseases; they caused more suffering and deaths than any other human activity in the history of medicine."

For more information on vaccinations and for a list of related organizations, check out http://thinktwice.com/global.htm. This web site boasts "the world's largest selection of uncensored information" on childhood and other vaccinations. Another site of interest with regard to vaccinations is http://www.garynull.com/marketplace/documents.asp.

CHAPTER 6

Toxic Metals

"Nearly all men die of their medicines, not of their disease."
Moliere

Toxic metals are minerals that are basically non-nutritive. They include heavy metals, some of which do not belong in the body at all and some which are only needed in minute amounts. When found there, they can do a great deal of harm by interfering with normal metabolic activity. Largely as a consequence of the pollution created by our modern, industrialized society, these metals are finding their way in increasing quantities into our bodies. Heavy metal poisoning is an often unrecognized cause of many physical and psychological disorders. The remaining pages of this chapter will identify the major toxic metals and their sources and present some ways to prevent and deal with the problem.

ALUMINUM

Technically speaking, aluminum is not a "heavy" metal, but it can be a toxic one if present in excessive amounts in the body. It is the most abundant of the metallic elements.

By now, I think most of us have gotten the word that it is not such a good idea to cook in aluminum vessels, for heat serves as a catalyst, causing the metal to be leached out of the vessel and into the food. The same thing happens if we cook food in aluminum foil. It is probably advisable to even avoid wrapping food for storage in aluminum foil. Although no heat is applied in this instance, the direct and prolonged contact of the foil with the food *could* cause a problem.

Anti-perspirants are also a source of aluminum toxicity. In this instance, the aluminum makes its way into the body through the skin. Repeated use of these products can cause a toxic build-up in the system, resulting in a swelling of lymph nodes under the arms. Read labels to determine the ingredients present in such products. A variety of non-toxic deodorants containing all natural ingredients is available in health food stores.

Aluminum soda cans are another source of the metal. Baking powders also are aluminum-containing. An exception is the Rumford brand, which has a cream of tartar base.

Finally, many antacids contain aluminum. Since Americans are now taking more antacids than any other type of medication, these products are viewed as a significant source of aluminum toxicity. Contrary to popular belief, it appears that the high incidence of stomach and duodenal ulcers in our society is not due primarily to over-acidity. Most of us are *deficient* in HCl (hydrochloric acid). Putrefaction of undigested protein may give the *appearance* of over-acidity, but ulcer formation itself is largely a result of the inability of the stomach to produce sufficient quantity of protective secretions that serve to prevent HCl from ulcerating surrounding tissue. This creates a terrain which is favorable for the survival of H. pylori, the microorganism recently found to be associated with ulcers.

Aluminum deposits in the brain have been highly correlated with Alzheimer's Disease. Toxicity can cause gastrointestinal irritation and convulsions. Rickets can also develop, as aluminum adversely affects calcium metabolism and therefore bone formation. Aluminum toxicity can also lead to nervousness, anemia, decreased liver and kidney function and muscle aches. Since calcium and magnesium are antagonistic to aluminum, adequate amounts of them in the diet will help reduce aluminum deposits.

*LEAD

Lead is one of the most toxic of the metal elements. This metabolic poison accumulates in the body, being absorbed directly from the blood into the tissues.

Lead is found in pesticides, fertilizers, some hair dyes and rinses, soft coal, cigarette smoke, cosmetics, pewter ware, and in pottery that was painted with lead-based glazes. Such glazes sold in the U.S have warning labels cautioning the consumer not to use them on items that will come into contact with food or beverages. We cannot be certain, however, about the glazes used in either antique or imported pottery. These may well contain lead and therefore should not be used to prepare or serve food items. Other sources of lead include lead-crystal dishes and glassware, lead-acid car batteries, some domestic and imported wines, contaminated bone meal supplements, lead pipes and lead *soldered* pipes.

Tap water is also a potential source of lead toxicity. It is estimated that one out of every five Americans served by public water systems consumes dangerous amounts of lead in their household water. Lead is nearly ubiquitous — particles of it have even been found in the snow in the Arctic!

While lead-based paints have been discontinued, older buildings and items of furniture still exist that had been coated with such paints. Chips of lead-based paint, when consumed by infants or toddlers, can have devastating effects, for children absorb lead up to ten times more efficiently than do adults.

Polluted air contains lead. In the U.S., the average is in excess of 35 mg. per day, higher in some cities and in industrial areas. Lead is inhaled into the body.

This metal is a poison that blocks enzymes at the cellular level. It interferes with blood formation and is stored in the bones. Symptoms of lead toxicity include abdominal pain, constipation, fatigue, weakness, paleness. High levels of lead in the body have also been linked with behavioral disorders and learning disabilities. Alexander Schauss *(Diet, Crime and Delinquency)* points to studies reporting that lead levels found to affect the behavior of school children were below 1 mg., the level most commonly considered toxic. He also points to medical journal articles linking lead levels with hyperactivity, a problem that affects a growing number of children in the U.S. Schauss suggests that lead toxicity is so widespread that all correctional facilities should routinely screen their inmates for it. Other possible symptoms of lead toxicity include diarrhea, anxiety, loss of appetite, tremors, seizures, gout, vertigo, insomnia and arthritis.

The following case history gives an idea of the potentially devastating effects of lead toxicity:

C.T., a thirty-three-year-old physician, became mentally ill with a diagnosis of paranoid schizophrenia. He was alcoholic and consuming large quantities of both drugs and alcohol while practicing medicine prior to entering a mental hospital. He responded poorly to treatment until a patient came to him asking for hair analysis. He had no prior knowledge of hair analysis, and, after looking into the matter, ordered a hair analysis not only for his patient but for himself. He discovered very high levels of lead in his own hair, four times the upper limit of what is considered to be acceptable in our culture and also elevated levels of cadmium, mercury and copper. The lead concentration was by far the highest into the toxic range. Following treatment ... his condition improved dramatically, and his symptoms of mental illness reverted to normal. He lost his craving for alcohol and had no further need for psychoactive drugs.(1)

NICKEL

Minute amounts of this metal are needed by the body to activate certain enzymes and to stabilize DNA and RNA. Excessive amounts of nickel, however, can cause serious problems in the body. These can include asthma, skin problems, cancer of the lungs and nasal passages, blood vessel damage, gingivitis, stomatitis, headaches, dizziness, convulsions, back pain and sinus conditions.

Nickel is found in jewelry, cosmetics, cold waving (permanents) and in welded joints. Also, the metal is used as a catalyst in the hydrogenation of oils and finds its way into the body in this manner. Additionally, it is widely used in dentistry. Though not widely known, nickel is a component of stainless steel. It can therefore enter the body through use of stainless steel cookware. Some amount of nickel is naturally occurring in buckwheat, oats, cabbage and legumes.

Research has shown that "every second or third person has some kind of nickel poisoning,"[2] according to Hanna Kroeger. She states that since opium is the antidote for nickel poisoning, and poppy seeds contain tiny amounts of opium, taking one tablespoon of these seeds twice daily may help to relieve toxicity symptoms.

*CADMIUM

Like lead, cadmium accumulates in the body. It replaces zinc in the liver and kidneys, and therefore high levels are found in zinc-deficient people.

Cadmium is found in cigarette smoke, paints, contaminated drinking water, galvanized pipes, oxide rusts, welded joints and in shellfish found near industrial shores. It was disclosed in the press early in 1988 that about 75% of U.S. seafood goes to market without being examined for impurities or tested for toxins. Exposés on filthy conditions in some seafood processing plants have caused closer scrutiny of the industry.

Additional sources of cadmium include nickel-cadmium batteries, plastics, fertilizers, fungicides, refined grains, rice, coffee, tea and soft drinks. Cadmium is also used in dentistry, in particular to impart the pink color to dentures.

Cadmium affects the heart, brain, blood vessels, the renal cortex of the kidneys, as well as the appetite and olfactory centers. Toxicity can give rise to hypertension, anemia, kidney and liver damage, decreased appetite and loss of smell. Cadmium toxicity weakens the immune system, as it causes decreased T cell production. It can also cause hair loss and dry, scaly skin.

*MERCURY

The toxicity level of mercury exceeds that of lead. This toxic metal is abundant in our environment, being found in our soil, water and food supply. Some grains are treated with methyl mercury chlorine bleaches.

Mercury is found in cosmetics, fluorescent lights, thermometers, barometers, fungicides, pesticides, fabric softeners, latex, printer's ink, some plastics, polishes, solvents, wood preservatives and hair dyes. Although not well-known, it has been used widely in indoor paints to retard mold. Unfortunately, disclosure of its presence in paints was not always required on the label. The EPA had considered regulating its use in paints in 1972, but was swayed against this action by representatives from the industry. Nonetheless, in the mid-1970s, DuPont, Glidden and Sherwin Williams voluntarily removed mercury from their paints. On 6/29/90, the EPA took more direct action and banned the use of mercury in all indoor latex paint. This action was prompted by the near-fatal poisoning of a 4-year old child in Michigan. This EPA ruling also requires that all exterior paints containing mercury be labeled.

Mercury is also found in fish from contaminated salt water and is used widely in dentistry as a major component of amalgams, metallic dental "fillings." This is a source of mercury toxicity that I will explore more thoroughly since it affects so many of us.

AMALGAMS

In the 16th century, mercury was widely used in medicine. It was found in ointments prescribed for treatment of syphilis. By the end of the 17th century, however, it was identified as a neurotoxicant. In 1685 mercury nitrate was used in France in the preparation of fur felt used in making hats. The workers inhaled the mercury vapors which affected their neurological systems — and that is the origin of the saying, "mad as a hatter," for mercury has an affinity for the brain.

The first metallic fillings appeared in the U.S. about 1820. Six years later, a silver paste, which was a combination of silver and mercury, was introduced. The silver came from smelted coins and so contained other metals as well; hence the name "amalgam." Previous to this time, the only filling material used had been gold, which few could afford.

The forerunner to the American Dental Association (ADA) was the American Society of Dental Surgeons. They stood in firm opposition to the use of mercury in dentistry because of its known toxic effects. However, in 1833, two brothers by the name of Crawcour set up practice in New York and exploited the use of amalgams by a rigorous and successful advertising campaign. They did a booming business, despite the fact that they had no formal training in dentistry. They were successful in creating a demand for the new filling material and attracted many patients previously associated with established legitimate dentists. This caused the dental profession and their society to retaliate, attacking the use of amalgams even more vigorously and eventually succeeding in forcing the Crawcours out of business.

For the next 25 years, the official stand of organized dentistry was solid opposition to the use of amalgam. There were some dissenting members, however, and in 1855, to end the conflicts within the Society, most of the resolutions that prohibited the use of amalgams were withdrawn. The internal conflict soon broke up the organization, however. Shortly thereafter, it was replaced by the ADA, which has always stood in favor of the use of dental amalgams.

New amalgam formulations were subsequently developed, and by 1870 the first organized movement in support of amalgams was launched. Claims were made that the material did not pose a health hazard. In 1900, Dr. G.V. Black succeeded in "perfecting" the dental amalgam. Soon thereafter, opposition to dental amalgams was rekindled, due largely to the work of Dr. Alfred Stock, a German chemistry professor. In an article written in 1926, he identified dental amalgam as a source of mercury vapor emissions that caused the following symptoms: tiredness, depression, irritability, vertigo, poor memory, mouth inflammations, diarrhea, loss of appetite and chroniccatarrhs. In 1939, Dr. Stock found the amalgam to be "an unstable alloy that continuously gave off mercury in the form of gas ions and abraded particles."(3)

It can be demonstrated by use of special equipment (the Jerome Mercury Vapor Analyzer) that the amount of mercury vapor being released from silver amalgams after the patient has chewed gum for ten minutes is excessive, often higher than mercury levels to which at-risk industrial workers are exposed. The implication here is that every time we chew (as in three meals per day), we are poisoning ourselves with mercury vapors, breathing in the fumes, as did the "mad hatters" of 17th century France. This is quite apart from any mercury particles that may be leached into the system through the tooth structure.

Today, amalgams are 50% mercury. The other 50% is a combination of silver, tin, copper and zinc. These dissimilar metals, placed in a solution of saliva, create conditions in the mouth conducive to the generation of electrical currents, for the saliva provides the needed electrolyte. The mouth therefore becomes a mini-generating plant. In some instances, people with enough dissimilar metal in their mouth can even pick up radio stations! This "oral galvanism" initiates a breakdown or corrosion of the amalgam fillings, increasing both the amount of mercury vapor and abraded particles that can be released in the mouth.

The ADA, in July of 1984, conceded that mercury is released from dental amalgams, but claimed that the amount released is too small to cause health problems *except in rare allergic individuals.* This remains their official position. In formulating this position, Sam Ziff and Dr. Michael Ziff tell us, the ADA seems to have "overlooked" studies which "demonstrate irrefutably that the percentage of allergy to amalgam and/or mercury can be as high as 44.3%."(4) They also tell us:

> In the more than 125 years that the ADA has been in existence, it has not funded one single research project proving the bio-compatibility or safety of dental amalgams in humans. There is conclusive scientific evidence showing a direct correlation between the numbers and surfaces of amalgam fillings and the mercury content of brain tissue. Scientific research has demonstrated that mercury, even in small amounts, can damage the brain, heart, lungs, liver, kidneys, thyroid gland, pituitary gland, adrenal glands, blood cells, enzymes, hormones and suppresses the body's immune system.
>
> In addition, mercury has been shown to pass the placental membrane in pregnant women and cause permanent damage to the brain of a developing baby.(5)

There is a growing public awareness regarding the hazards posed by mercury-containing amalgams. A class action suit has been filed in Canada as a result of this. More than one such suit is in the works in the U.S. as well.

Dr. David G. Williams tells us that "while interior paints were limited to 300 ppm and exterior ones to 2,000 ppm, maximum limits for dental fillings have never been set [and] silver amalgam fillings contain 500,000 ppm of mercury!"[6]

Dentists, with their constant exposure to mercury, have a higher rate of suicide than any other occupation (remember the mad hatters?). It is also interesting that cadavers of dentists showed 800 times more mercury than those of non-dentists.[7]

There was a time when gold fillings were the only alternative to amalgams. That time has passed. Gold is still available, but new composite and ceramic materials have been developed, which are not only cheaper but may be preferable. Although gold is relatively biocompatible, the type used in dentistry is an alloy, mixed usually with palladium, copper or cobalt. The actual percentage of gold can vary from 2-92%. Palladium is generally considered to be a safe dental material. It is not. It is a strong allergen. The different palladium alloys (over 100) have caused serious adverse side effects, including dying teeth, cardiac arrhythmia and facial paralysis. It is more difficult to rid the body of palladium than to get rid of amalgam, for it cannot be chelated. Also, palladium-poisoned people tend to be electrosensitive.[8]

The newer tooth-colored materials are referred to variously as "bonded resin ceramics," "composite resins" or just "composites." These materials are demonstrated to have a higher degree of biocompatibility than the amalgams. It is imperative to realize, however, that not all of these materials are compatible with the biochemistry of all people. There has been little research regarding the side effects and overall safety of composites. Therefore, compatibility testing of all dental materials, prior to placement in the mouth, is essential. Specialized blood tests (Clifford and Huggins) are available to establish biocompatibility of dental materials. ElectroDermal Screening (see chapter 12) can also be used for this purpose and yields highly reliable results. I prefer it to the blood testing. Simple muscle testing can also be used but with less quantitative (and sometimes less reliable) results.

"Today's composites show better durability than amalgam. There is some concern, however, about the effects of their undeclared components. Also of concern are reported side effects, chief of which are allergies."(9)   Unbelievably, "X-ray opacity in composites has been achieved by adding various heavy metal fillers, some of which are toxic, others *radioactive.*"(10)   So, while composites. appear to be less toxic than amalgam, they, too, can be quite hazardous and should be selected with caution.

You are not likely to be fortunate enough to find a dentist who will actually *recommend* replacing your amalgams with non-metallic material due to the ADA's official stand on the subject. For that same reason, insurance will not cover the cost of replacement unless you somehow manage to demonstrate that you are one of the "rare" allergic individuals. The ADA's insistence on the safety of amalgam, despite overwhelming evidence to the contrary, may have a huge amount to do with the fact that they have been the primary patent holder of mercury amalgam.(11) Each amalgam filling placed had been money in their pockets!

Amalgam is also used as filling material in root canals. Dr. Weston Price, former Director of Research for the American Dental Association, spent 35 years researching the link between root canal filled teeth and heart, kidney and uterine disease, as well as disorders of the nervous and endocrine systems. He demonstrated that damage to these organs results from seepage of toxins from the root canal filled teeth. Read *Root Canal Cover Up* by George Meinig, DDS, for details on the problems posed by root canals. These problems are also touched upon in my book, *Beyond Amalgam: The Hidden Health Hazard Posed by Jawbone Cavitations.* This book deals with the subject of jawbone cavitations, a condition caused not only by root canals but also standard extractions (especially of wisdom teeth). This condition is widespread, though under-diagnosed and can be the unsuspected cause of many systemic health problems. A cavitation is not the same thing as a cavity. It is a hole in the bone (not the tooth), caused most frequently by faulty extraction technique. Failure of the dentist to remove the ligament which attaches the bone to the tooth, and to properly clean out the socket, results in the formation of a hidden hole or pocket in the bone. This hollowed out area becomes a breeding ground for microbes and their toxins. The net result is bone infection (osteomyelitis) and bone death (osteonecrosis). It is a very serious and widespread (though seldom recognized) condition for which we presently have no cure, though surgical removal of necrotic bone does appear to be necessary. The condition is the hidden cause of many seemingly unrelated health problems throughout the body, for there is a relationship between each tooth in the mouth and the various organs.

For more information on the subject of mercury amalgam toxicity and other dental issues, and/or the names of dentists who practice mercury-free dentistry in your area, contact DAMS (Dental Amalgam Mercury Survivors) at 1-800-311-6265 (www.dams.cc).

Mercury can cause cell destruction, block transport of sugars and increase permeability of potassium. High levels interfere with enzyme activity. Toxicity symptoms, in addition to those already mentioned, can include emotional disturbances, recurring infections, blood changes, chewing and swallowing difficulties, arthritis, dermatitis, dizziness, gum disease, hair loss, insomnia, muscle weakness, excessive salivation, loss of pain sensation and convulsions.

Due to the health and environmental hazards posed by mercury, several countries have either banned the use of amalgam fillings, greatly limited their use or issued warnings regarding their use. Countries taking such action include Germany, Austria, Sweden, Norway, Switzerland, Denmark, Holland, France, Canada and Japan. Japanese Dental Schools, in fact, are no longer teaching the use of mercury.

The toxic metals not only damage the body directly but also indirectly in that they "encourage the transmutation of other elements into themselves, and thereby increase the levels of toxicity of those elements."(12)

DIAGNOSING AND TREATING
METAL TOXICITY

Heavy metal toxicity often goes unrecognized and untreated, largely because symptoms are not correctly identified by medical doctors. The hair analysis mentioned earlier in our discussion of lead poisoning is not generally known to, nor used by, M.Ds. It is more likely to be employed by a nonmedical physician, a D.C. or a N.D. (A small sample of untreated hair, usually taken from the nape of the neck, is used in hair analysis.) Such tests will not necessarily give an accurate indication of the amount of nutritive minerals present in the cell system, but they often do accurately reflect the presence and concentrations of toxic metals. Analysis of urine (for porphyrin content) and fecal samples can also help reveal the presence of metals in the body. Excessive levels of the heavy metals can be reduced through either oral or intravenous chelation therapy and/or through the use of homeopathic preparations.

It is beyond the scope of this book to describe the practice of homeopathy. Suffice it to say that it is one of the oldest of the healing arts and is practiced widely outside of the U.S. It involves the use of highly diluted natural medicines and works on the principle or law of similars (like attracts like). Its effectiveness is not in the action of its physical substance, for there is little to none present in the remedies, but rather in the *affinity of frequency* that it has for the condition being treated.

A chelating agent, as previously mentioned, is a substance that binds with a mineral, facilitating its transport either into or out of the body. Chelated minerals are bound with a chelating agent, usually an amino acid, which helps carry them into the cell system. Chelation therapy involves utilizing the same principle to *remove* toxic metals from the body.

Intravenous chelation therapy serves as sort of a chemical "roto rooter" to clean out clogged arteries. It is a process that has been used in the treatment of heavy metal poisoning in the U.S. since 1948 and for hardening of the arteries since 1952. EDTA (ethylene diamine tetraacetic acid), a synthetic amino acid, is the most commonly used chemical chelating agent. Penacillamine is another chemical chelating agent that has been traditionally used. These, however, are potentially toxic. Intravenous chelation therapy is costly and involves repeated sessions of IV infusion. Treatments are generally given in segments of 12, and a total of 30-50 sessions is typically needed. The procedure is used not only in the treatment of heavy metal poisoning and atherosclerosis but also in stroke, kidney stones, arthritis and bursitis and a number of eye diseases. Intravenous chelation therapy is not widely accepted nor practiced in medical circles, for it is a controversial alternative treatment. It is certainly a viable alternative to coronary by-pass surgery, however! Please bear in mind that the purpose of chelation therapy is to remove inorganic mineral deposits from the body. These can be removed, only to be redeposited, however, if the physician and his patient are not aware of dietary and lifestyle patterns that cause build-up of such minerals. Also, some nutritive minerals are removed in the IV chelation process. Care should be taken therefore to replace these. It should be noted that EDTA chelation therapy, while used to treat mercury toxicity, is not particularly effective in this regard, for research (by Foulkes and Bergman) has shown that it is unable to disassociate the metal from cell membranes.

Specific nutrients, notably vitamin C, N-Acetylcysteine, alpha-lipoic acid and vitamin E, play an important role in ridding the body of heavy metals, either by directly chelating them or by supporting the body in its own efforts to remove the poisonous metals. Oral chelation is possible with the use of such nutrients, either in whole food or extracted form.

The chemicals DMPS and DMSA are used widely by physicians to chelate mercury, as they flush the metal out of the tissues and into the urine. These should be used with extreme care and only under medical supervision where excretion levels can be monitored, however. Dr. Deborah Baker (www.y2khealthanddetox.com) warns about the inappropriate and indiscriminate widespread use of these potentially harmful chemical chelating agents. DMPS, she tells us, is "a combination of propane, sulfonic acid and thiols. Both propane and sulfonic acid are difficult for us to metabolize. Therefore, allergic reactions, autoimmune responses and mercury redistribution are of great concern." There are numerous potential side effects of DMPS treatment, including *mercury poisoning,* as the metal can be re-distributed throughout the body, causing significant organ damage and a host of symptoms.

DMSA appears to be somewhat safer than DMPS but should still be administered under medical supervision. The patient should be tested for sensitivity to both of these chelating agents before either is administered. While DMPS acts like a sulfa drug in the body, DMSA, an orally administed chemical, does not. It has a base of succinic acid and is the only chemical chelator known to cross the blood-brain barrier. It can therefore help remove mercury from the brain. Dr. Baker recommends starting *very slowly,* one week on, one week off, replacing the nutritive minerals that are removed along with the mercury.

Certain foods, notably those high in the sulfur-containing amino acids, can be used to help chelate heavy metals, such as mercury, from the body. Those foods rich in these amino acids include beans, eggs, onions and garlic. Another natural chelating agent is algin, found abundantly in kelp and other sea vegetables such as chlorella and spirulina. Care should be taken when using these algaes, however, that they are not themselves contaminated with heavy metals from polluted waters. Cilantro, Chinese parsley, was found by a Japanese medical doctor, Omura, to effectively move mercury and other heavy metals out of the cells. It is used as a primary chelator by many alternative doctors today.

The decision of whether to use chemical chelating agents, homeopathic remedies, nutritional supplements or natural foods will depend upon the severity of the toxicity and the judgment of the physician. Homeopathy is often the treatment of choice initially when the patient is very ill, and detoxification pathways are blocked.

Ideally, screening for heavy metal toxicity would be a routine part of any annual check-up, given the prevalence of these pollutants in our society and the likelihood that they will find their way into our bodies. Once the problem is identified, appropriate treatment can be initiated.

There is much we can do to avoid heavy metal poisoning and/or to alleviate the body's burden of inorganic minerals. I recommend switching to a pure water source, eating whole, unprocessed foods, having amalgam fillings replaced with biologically compatible non-metallic materials (after cavitations are ruled out/treated) and avoiding the ingestion of inorganic minerals in supplement form. In addition, we can familiarize ourselves with the sources of heavy metal toxicity and avoid or minimize exposure to such contaminants.

----

*There has been no nutritive need established for these metals (lead, cadmium, mercury).

CHAPTER 7

The Effect of Light
Upon Health

*"Where the sun does not go,
the doctor goes."*
Old Italian Saying

There are two aspects of light with which we need concern ourselves: intensity and quality. Even the brightest artificial light is not nearly as intense as sunlight. In fact, it is ten times brighter in the shade than it is in the average artificially lighted indoor environment. Dr. Zane Kime, M.D., *(Sunlight)* tells us that this aspect of light affects our health, citing a rabbit study which showed that those animals, when kept in a fairly dim light, were susceptible to cancer. An increase in light, however, resulted in a *decrease* in cancer.

The pineal gland, located in the center of the skull just above the eyes, reacts to sunlight. This gland produces the hormone melatonin, which helps regulate our internal clocks. The pineal gland seems to have a regulatory effect upon other glands as well, and therefore its ability to initiate (in darkness) and shut off (in light) the production of melatonin is critical to the entire body.

It has been found that the majority of people over 40 in the U.S. have calcified or atrophied pineal glands. Such calcified glands are no longer able to regulate melatonin secretion. A lack of melatonin production causes estrogen release. Over-abundance of estrogen in the system is correlated with a high incidence of female type cancers. We find, however, that in the developing countries, where women have normally functioning pineal glands, there is a low incidence of breast and uterine cancers. Their pineal glands function normally due to adequate exposure to natural sunlight during the day and total darkness at night. An imbalance of both estrogen and melatonin results from interference with day/night cycles, which can come from artificial lights.

Dr. Kime cites Russian studies which showed that laboratory animals developed "much less cancer" when given ultraviolet light (UV) by means of special sun lamps. This discovery was particularly interesting because it had been the researchers intent to *induce* cancer through the use of the UV lamps. They found, much to their surprise, however, that it was not the animals living under the UV lights but those under the *fluorescent* lights that developed the cancer!

It has become a popular belief that sunlight causes cancer. While *overexposure* to the ionizing UV rays of the sun can cause tissue damage via production of free radicals and consequent development of cancer or other degenerative diseases, a certain amount of daily exposure to sunlight is not only harmless but is, in fact, necessary for the maintenance of health. It was discovered almost a century ago that sunlight has an important role to play in the functioning of the immune system. In fact, one physician won the Nobel Prize for showing how sunlight could heal tuberculosis. Other researchers demonstrated the sun's effectiveness in treating strep, staph and viral infections.

The UV-C or far-UV rays have bactericidal qualities. They are, however, the most harmful of the UV rays and are absorbed by the ozone. The UV-B or mid-UV rays also have the ability to kill bacteria and other microorganisms. They play a role in calcium absorption as well. The UV-A or near-UV rays induce the tanning response. This is the most healthful part of the UV portion of the light spectrum and is necessary for photosynthesis.

When sunlight falls on the skin, the immune system is stimulated to increase the number of white blood cells, specifically the lymphocytes. The lymphocytes produce gamma globin and interferon, immune serums which protect from infection.

Because of its known bactericidal effect, sunlight was once widely used as a treatment for infectious disease. However, it fell into disuse when antibiotic therapy became popular. Today's medical students are no longer taught that sunlight stimulates the immune system. Instead, the harmful effects of over-exposure to UV are stressed.

Apart from killing bacteria, sunlight has other known benefits. Sunbathing has been demonstrated to lower blood pressure and keep it lowered for up to 4 to 5 days after exposure to the sun. Sunlight on the skin increases the amount of oxygen in the tissues and bloodstream. The oxygen, as we know, is needed in combination with glucose to produce ATP to fuel the electrical generators of the body. Lack of oxygen at the cellular level produces conditions conducive to impaired immunity and disease development. Sunlight also lowers blood sugar and cholesterol levels.

If all of this is so, if sunlight has so many *beneficial* qualities, why then is it getting so much bad press lately? Why has it become linked so strongly with cancer in the minds of most? My belief is that, under certain conditions, the sun can serve as a catalyst in the development of cancer, but under optimal conditions its protective benefits are apparent. The "optimal conditions" of which I speak are basically adherence to a healthy lifestyle and dietary patterns, coupled with a pollution-free environment. Such conditions are practically non-existent in our culture today. But in certain more "primitive" ones, where these conditions are met, cancer is unknown, despite heavy exposure to sunlight without the "protection" of sunglasses and sunscreen!

The high incidence of cancer in our culture has a lot more to do with our lifestyle and environment than it has to do with the sun, whose rays are universally distributed and yet apparently nourish some while seeming to harm others. In looking at why sunlight *appears* to cause cancer, let us turn our attention to the subject of fats and what causes them to become rancid.

There are three conditions under which fats turn rancid: exposure to *heat, oxygen* and *light.* Our tissues provide the heat and oxygen. When we consume fat (or rub oil on our skin) and then expose ourselves to sunlight, thus satisfying the third condition, we can be assured that the fat we have consumed, as well as the oil on our skin, will turn rancid (although chances are very good that it was already rancid). Rancid oil gives rise to the development of free radicals, those renegade chemical fragments so heavily implicated in degenerative disease development. Ionizing radiation can also give rise to free radical production. Therefore, it has been assumed that cancer formation results from free radicals produced by the sun's ionizing UV rays. Could it be that it results more predominantly from the free radicals produced by rancid oils taken internally and used externally?

There is a group of nutrients known as "antioxidants" that serves to prevent rancidity. These nutrients include vitamins A, C, E, the minerals selenium and zinc and the sulfur-containing amino acids. Many of these nutrients are removed from food in the refining process. Vitamins A and E, being fat-soluble, are rendered unavailable to the system when mineral oil (an ingredient in sun tan oils) or hydrogenated fats are used. Vitamin C, as a water-soluble vitamin, is rapidly depleted under stress. Since we Americans consume many refined foods, including hydrogenated oil, and are under a lot of stress, we tend to be deficient in antioxidant nutrients. Therefore, fats that we consume have little protection from rancidity. A study done at Baylor Medical College in Texas showed that animals exposed to ten times the normal sunlight did not develop cancer when they were given *extra amounts of antioxidants.* The antioxidants prevent cancer by guarding against rancidity. So, perhaps our society's proneness to cancer has more to do with dietary deficiency than with "dangers" from the sun. It is plain to see how the sun can serve as a catalyst to accelerate rancidity of oils and fats, which, in turn, can lead to cancer. However, the process *began* as a consequence of dietary inadequacy.

Antioxidant nutrients, which guard against rancidity and subsequent free radical formation, are found naturally and abundantly in whole foods. Once again, food processing is found to play a major role in disease causation due to the nutrient deficiencies it causes. An unrefined diet is highly recommended for protection from cancer, regardless of sun exposure.

The subject of light quality is addressed in the work of Dr. John Ott who has done extensive research on the effects of light on biological systems. His work and writings address the relationship between the wavelength components (colors) of natural sunlight and our physical and mental health. Dr. Ott has experimented with what is now known as "time-lapse" photography since he was in high school over 60 years ago. As a photobiologist, he developed the techniques that made it possible to observe the maturation of plants in minutes, as viewed in some of Walt Disney's nature films. In the process of doing this work, he found that, under certain conditions, flowers refused to bloom. In filming one of Disney's episodes, Ott observed that pumpkin seeds would not mature properly under fluorescent lights but thrived if a UV light source was added.

Dr. Ott observed that light affected animal life in a variety of interesting ways. Fish, he found, stopped laying eggs when placed under 40 watt fluorescent tubes. When exposure to this light was reduced to eight hours, egg-laying resumed, but the offspring produced under the pink fluorescents were all female! Reproduction normalized under full-spectrum lighting conditions. "Full-spectrum" lighting is sunlight or an artificial light designed to mimic sunlight in terms of its wavelength composition. The graph below shows the wavelength or color distribution found in full-spectrum lights, both artificial and natural:

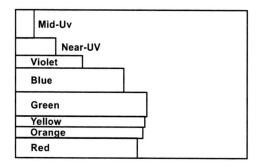

In contrast to the full-spectrum profile, commonly used artificial lighting presents a distortion of wavelength patterns. Note on the graphs below the unevenness of wavelengths in the incandescent and cool-white fluorescent lights.

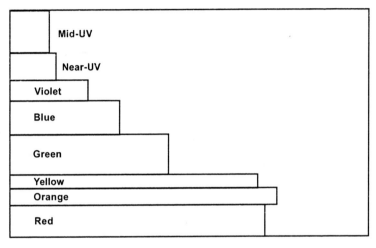

Incadescent

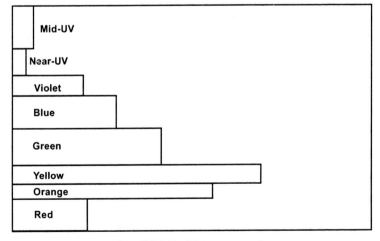

Cool White Flourescent

Notice especially the reduced amount of near-UV in the artificial lights. The incandescent light produces its maximum energy in the infrared wavelengths, while the cool-white fluorescent is disproportionately high in the yellow wavelength. Repeated exposure to such light produces a condition that Ott terms *"malillumination."* Light influences many physiological functions including our metabolic rate, respiration rate, blood pressure, liver, kidney and pancreas functions, immune response and maintenance of biological rhythms. Emotional stability is also affected. Two to three percent of the middle-to-northern latitude population of the U.S. are affected by a condition known as "Seasonal Affective Disorder." This condition is characterized by severe depression and fatigue at the onset of winter and is related to diminished exposure to sunlight. Phototherapy (light therapy) has proved effective in treatment of Seasonal Affective Disorder if it is sufficiently intense and is administered for a sufficient duration of time. The quality of the light is, as you might suppose, an important variable in determining the success of phototherapy. Studies conducted at the Department of Psychiatry at the University Hospital in Vancouver, Canada, involving 11 patients during the winter of 1988-89, showed that UV light was more effective than both UV-blocked and dim conditions in treating Seasonal Affective Disorder.

Full-spectrum light has also been used to treat psoriasis, neonatal jaundice, herpes simplex infections and skin inflammation. Light can help regulate the rhythms of the body. As mentioned, it has been shown to reduce high blood pressure and cholesterol and to stimulate the immune system. Full-spectrum light regulates hormonal secretion and decreases work fatigue and eye strain which can result from artificial lighting conditions.

Prolonged exposure to fluorescent lights can cause a number of undesirable effects including eyestrain, headaches, insomnia, irritability, hyperactivity, fatigue and even increased dental caries. And yet, these lights are routinely used in nearly all of our country's offices and institutions, including schools and hospitals. In 1980, Dr. Fritz Hollowich conducted a study that monitored endocrine changes resulting from illumination by cool-white fluorescent lights vs. full-spectrum lighting. He found that exposure to the fluorescents resulted in release of stress hormones (ACTH and cortisol), whereas no such reaction occured with full-spectrum lights.[1] Based on the research of Hollowich and others, Germany banned the use of the cool-white fluorescent bulb in hospitals and other medical facilities.

Incandescent bulbs, as previously mentioned, produce their maximum energy in the red end of the spectrum. Constant exposure to such distorted lighting can cause problems according to microscopic time-lapse studies of animal cells in tissue culture. In such studies, Dr. Ott found variations in growth patterns with different color filters. *A red filter consistently weakened and ruptured cell walls.* Ott also found that no mitosis (cell division) occurred with three or more hours of exposure of cells to either red or blue light. Mitosis only took place under full-spectrum (white) lighting conditions. Ott also found he could increase the metabolic activity of cells or even kill them by changing lighting conditions.

Not only is the physical condition of an organism affected by light but so is the mental condition. Behaviors of laboratory animals will change greatly as lighting conditions are changed. Researchers have long known it is necessary to remove a male rat from his cage in the laboratory before his pregnant mate gives birth; otherwise he will cannibalize the newborn rats. However, it has been found that under full-spectrum lighting conditions this does not occur. In a sunlit environment, or one approximating it artificially with full-spectrum bulbs, papa rat will actually nurture his offspring!

To a lesser degree, humans seem to be similarly affected by light. Experiments carried out in 1986 in a classroom at Green Street Elementary School in Brattleboro, Vermont, and reported in *The Lancet* on 11/21/87, showed that children attending classes in a room illuminated by full-spectrum lights took fewer days off from school due to illness than other students. In the 1970s, Dr. Ott set up a study in Sarasota, Florida where he resides. He introduced full-spectrum lighting into a classroom at Gocio Elementary School and found that such lighting improved not only general attendance but also the behavior of hyperactive children. Their learning ability and concentration were also enhanced. Further studies have confirmed these benefits.

In his research, John Ott found the key to the link between light and health. That key is in the act of light entering the eye. When light hits the retina, necessary glandular stimulation occurs. The pituitary, pineal and hypothalamus glands are activated. Light causes the pineal gland to temporarily suspend melatonin production. Lack of exposure to full-spectrum light prevents the necessary suspension of melatonin production and can lead to glandular exhaustion. Under artificial lighting conditions, adequate glandular stimulation fails to take place largely due to lack of the necessary

UV portion of the spectrum. Glass has been found to screen out UV wavelengths. The glass found in household and automobile windows, eyeglasses and sunglasses blocks out this vital UV — and, far from "protecting" us, can make us vulnerable to disease due to lack of glandular stimulation. Eyeglasses and contact lenses block 92% of incoming UV radiation. Sunglasses can be particularly harmful due to their tint, which distorts the color spectrum. Recall the effects of red filters upon cell growth, and forego the rose-colored or other tinted glasses. Dr. Ott suggests that if sunglasses must be worn, a neutral gray color be selected, for it will at least cut down on all wavelengths equally. It is recommended that any sunglasses be removed periodically to allow the rays of the sun to act upon the retina, facilitating necessary glandular stimulation. To reap the benefit of sunlight entering the eyes, it is not necessary to situate oneself in bright light. The shade will do nicely. Remember: It's ten times brighter there than it is inside.

Dr. Ott tells an interesting story regarding sunglasses in his book *Health and Light.* Engaged in conversation at a dinner party with Albert Schweitzer's daughter, he was questioned as to the possible reasons why some members of a Congolese tribe had suddenly developed cancer when the disease had been previously unknown to the tribe. Speculating as to possible causes, he asked if houses with glass windows had recently been constructed. No. Had artificial lighting been introduced? No. Then, he half jokingly inquired as to whether the natives had been wearing sunglasses. Yes!! The glasses had been introduced into the tribe and were worn as a status symbol by the natives who frequently wore nothing but a loin cloth and the sunglasses!

Despite research supporting the beneficial effects of full-spectrum lighting and the damaging effects of artificial light, the majority of our institutions continue to use the standard fluorescent bulbs. Why? For one thing, we have operating once again the element of vested interest. General Electric does not concede that light serves any but a visual function in humans. This huge and influential company does not recognize the effect of light on health, a link which Ott has devoted his life to establishing. For a company like GE to adopt full-spectrum lighting would be tantamount to admitting the inadequacies of the fluorescent and incandescent lights presently being used. Where then does one turn for full-spectrum lights other than to the sun?

In the late 1960s, Duro-Test, the fourth largest lighting manufacturer in the country and the largest independent manufacturer, began marketing a full-spectrum fluorescent tube known as the "Vita-Lite" under Ott's direction. It was this Vita-Lite that was used in the classroom studies in Florida. It was also used in a Boston study conducted at a home for the elderly. Here it was demonstrated that the rate of calcium absorption increases with the use of full-spectrum lighting. While numerous favorable results were achieved with the use of this light, Dr. Ott was not satisfied with its performance, claiming that its cathodes gave off low level x-rays, and that after about six months the lights failed to give off UV radiation. He claimed that when he approached Duro-Test, the company was not interested in correcting these problems. They maintain, however, that they did correct them. Nonetheless, Ott went on to produce his own product, the "Ott Light System." It is actually an entire lighting fixture rather than just a fluorescent tube. To be full-spectrum, lights must contain the UV or invisible part of the spectrum as well as the visible part, for it is the lack of UV radiation in the commonly used artificial lights that seems to be the main cause of health problems associated with them.

John Ott's work on the biological effects of light is now being carried on by Fred Mendelsohn, president of Environmental Lighting Concepts (Tampa, Florida) and Executive Director of Environmental Health and Light Research Institute, an organization founded by Ott which has done much to enhance public awareness regarding the beneficial effects of full-spectrum light (www.ott-lite.com).

Mendelsohn developed the phototherapy units used so effectively in treatment of Seasonal Affective Disorders. He developed these units in consultation with physicians at Johns Hopkins University. It was largely because of this work that Ott selected him to carry on his light research.

Given the information presented in this chapter, the notion of protecting ourselves from the rays of the sun by wearing sunglasses that wrap half way around our heads and enveloping ourselves in a cocoon of rancid sun tan oil becomes ludicrous....

Just as exposure to full-spectrum light during daytime hours is necessary for health maintenance, so too is avoidance of artificial light during sleeping hours. Such illumination inhibits melatonin production by the pineal gland and may throw off the estrogen balance in the body, increasing the risk for certain types of cancer. It is desirable therefore to sleep in total darkness. Dispense with night lights.

Exposing the body to full-spectrum light is analogous to taking a multiple vitamin, hoping that it will fill any unidentified nutritional gap. If you know what vitamin is lacking, you can supply it alone and have a more specific effect. So, too, with the wavelengths of light. If you know which one is deficient, it can be supplied in the form of a single color. This is the basis of color therapy, where different conditions are treated with different colors.

COLOR THERAPY

Directing light that has been filtered through colored gels at specific body parts is a color therapy technique that has a fascinating history and has yielded some impressive results. The pioneering work on this therapy was done by the late Dinshah P. Ghadaiali (known simply as "Dinshah") who migrated from India to America in 1911. He had a background in physics, chemistry, mathematics and electricity. Dinshah's system of color therapy came to be known as Spectro-Chrome. For his work in this area, he was awarded honorary medical degrees.

One of Dinshah's most notable and enthusiastic students had been Kate Baldwin, M.D. For 23 years, Dr. Baldwin had been senior surgeon at Philadelphia Woman's Hospital. During her last three years there, she used Spectro-Chrome methods, both at the hospital and in her private practice. On 10/12/26, she presented a paper on Spectro-Chrome at a clinical meeting of the section on Eye, Ear, Nose and Throat Diseases of the Medical Society of the State of Pennsylvania. An abstract of that paper was printed in the April 1927 edition of the *Atlantic Medical Journal.*

In her paper, she observed that each earth element "gives off a characteristic color wave:" Hydrogen, red and oxygen, blue. "{Give} the color representing the lacking elements, and the body will, through its radioactive forces, appropriate them and so restore the normal balance." She considered color to be "the simplest and most accurate therapeutic measure yet developed" and frankly stated that after 37 years of medical and surgical practice she could "produce quicker and more accurate results with colors than with any or all other methods combined — and with less strain on the patient." She added that "In many cases, the functions have been restored after the classical remedies have failed." While she conceded that surgery was necessary in some cases, she felt that results would be "quicker and better if color is used before and after [an] operation." Dr. Baldwin gave an exhaustive list of medical conditions successfully treated with Spectro-Chrome. These included sprains and bruises, septic conditions, cardiac lesions, asthma, hay fever, pneumonia, eye conditions and burns, as well as all sorts of trauma. With regard to burns, Dr. Baldwin had this to say:

> In such cases, the burning sensation caused by the destructive forces may be counteracted in from 20 to 30 minutes, and it does not return. True burns are caused by the destructive action of the red side of the spectrum, hydrogen predominating. Apply oxygen by the use of the blue side of the spectrum, and much will be done to relieve the nervous strain. The healing processes are rapid and the resulting tissues soft and flexible.(2)

Kate Baldwin felt so strongly about the efficacy of Spectro-Chrome that she wrote in a letter to a colleague, "I would close my office tonight never to reopen if I could not use Spectro-Chrome."

Despite glowing testimonials from people like Dr. Baldwin, Dinshah met with many obstacles in his work — a fire in the Institute's main building in 1945, which destroyed much of his work, fines and injunctions issued by the FDA that ordered him to "surrender for destruction" all books relating to Spectro-Chrome.

Dinshah died in 1966, but his work lives on in a limited way through the Dinshah Health Society (100 Dinshah Dr., Malaga, NY 08328 or on the web at www.wj.net/dinshah). The suppression of his work is reminiscent of the suppression of Béchamp and Rife's work. Like Rife, Dinshah was using frequency to heal. Such work was, and is, a threat to the medical-pharmaceutical monopoly that would have us believe that healing is accomplished only through chemical means.

At the same time that Dinshah was developing Sprectro-Chrome, Dr. Harry Riley Spitler, a M.D. with four doctorates (including one in optometry), was developing the science of Syntonics. Syntonics involves delivery of the various colors through the eyes — the most direct and quickest route to the centers of the brain which control all bodily functions. While Dinshah worked with a set of 12 color filter, Spitler used up to 31 different color combinations, treating patients according to their physical and emotional make-up, as well as their constitutional type. In 1933, he established the College of Syntonic Optometry, which defined Syntonics as "that branch of ocular science dealing with selected portions of the visible spectrum."

The effects of Syntonics go beyond visual improvement. It reflexively affects the entire body, integrating the nervous system and bringing major bodily functions into balance with the environment. Jacob Liberman, O.D., Ph.D., brought Syntonics to the attention of the public in 1991 with publication of his important book, *Light: Medicine of the Future.* In it, he points out that Syntonics can significantly enlarge the size of the visual field, resulting in enhanced learning ability and overall health improvement.

Today we are seeing a resurgence in color therapy, sound therapy, magnetic therapy and many forms of electrical therapy, all aimed at affecting the subtle energy body of man, which, in turn, will impact the physical body and its chemical constituents. These are, indeed, higher forms of healing, for they work with the forces that give rise to and impact the physical body rather than manipulating the bodily processes directly.

❧ CHAPTER 8 ❧

Electromagnetic Pollution

"If you feed a cold, you'll have to starve a fever."
Hippocrates

Those of us who are old enough to remember will recall the controversy in the 1960s regarding x-ray emissions from color television sets. Dr. John Ott, the photobiologist whose work was described in the last chapter, was among the first to identify this problem and attempt to correct it. He had read in the November 6, 1964 edition of *Time* magazine an article entitled "Those Tired Children." It described a case of 30 children, all manifesting the same set of mysterious symptoms, all of whom had watched TV 27-50 hours per week. Symptoms subsided in those children who followed the doctor's advice of eliminating television viewing from their daily regimen. The article went on to speculate as to the reasons why the excessive television viewing would cause such symptoms as nervousness, continuous fatigue, headache, loss of sleep and vomiting. The speculation emphasized such psychological considerations as over-stimulation from program content. No consideration was given to radiation leakage from the sets – except by Ott as he read the article. He subsequently set up tests using bean plants and later rats to test his hypothesis and found that growth rate, behavior and reproduction were all adversely affected by prolonged TV exposure such as that described in the article.

These effects were linked to x-ray radiation from the sets, for control groups exposed to sets whose picture tubes were lead-shielded were not so affected. On the basis of his findings, Ott expressed the opinion that hyperactivity in children, which has become a widespread problem, may well be due to the exposure to radiation from TV sets. When Ott reported the results of his findings to two large television manufacturing companies, one did not respond, and the other, RCA, conducted their own studies, finding their sets to be perfectly safe. Their director of research was quoted as saying, "It is utterly impossible for any TV set today to give off any harmful x-rays."

Soon thereafter, General Electric recalled thousands of their color sets due to x-ray emissions which they claimed were "not enough to cause concern." Later, the U.S. Surgeon General's office announced that the issue of x-ray emission was an industry-wide problem and not confined to GE. Radiation levels as high as 1.6 *million* times the accepted safety level were measured by the National Committee on Radiation Protection. This led to the passage of the 1968 Radiation Control Act, setting limits on radiation emissions from TV sets. However, government standards were considered by many (including consumer advocate, Ralph Nader) to be too low to assure full protection. Since 1968, TV x-ray emission standards have been lowered eight times. However, it appears that x-ray radiation *down to the zero level* penetrates body tissues, causing subtle but harmful effects. The closer to the TV set we sit, the greater the potential damage, and yet, at a distance of as much as 15 feet, reproduction was disturbed in Ott's rats.

X-rays are a form of ionizing radiation. When radiation strikes other material, it transfers its energy. At certain levels, it has enough energy to knock electrons out of atoms. This "ionizing" effect breaks up the molecular structure and can blow the DNA molecule apart. X-rays, gamma rays (used in food irradiation) and some UV radiation are ionizing forms of radiation that give rise to the creation of free radicals that, in turn, are linked to symptoms associated with aging and degenerative disease.

The electromagnetic spectrum looks like this:

↑ **Cosmic Rays**
   Gamma Rays
   X-rays
↑ **Ultraviolet (UV)**
   Visible Light
   Infrared
↑ **Microwaves**
   Radio Waves
   Extremely Low Frequencies (ELF)

Energy increases as we move from the bottom to the top of this spectrum. The higher the frequency, the shorter the waves. Below a certain UV level, radiation has a non-ionizing effect — i.e., it is too weak to rip electrons away from atoms, but at some frequencies it can still shake up matter and create heat, as is produced by microwaves, which are actually very short radio waves.

Radiation in the "Extremely Low Frequency" (ELF) range is generally considered to be below 300 hertz or cycles per second. Such low level magnetic fields were traditionally thought to have no effect upon biological systems. Research has shown, however, that such effects do exist and can range from extremely beneficial to absolutely lethal, depending upon the specific frequency and other conditions. Our 60 cycle household current falls into the ELF range and unfortunately this has been established to be a frequency that does not produce beneficial effects on living organisms.

Dr. Robert 0. Becker, M.D., did research with mice in the 1970s to ascertain the effect of 60 cycle current. He exposed the animals for 30 days to a strength of this frequency equivalent to that found in the area near high voltage power lines and found that they demonstrated hormonal, weight and body chemistry changes similar to those exhibited by animals under chronic stress. By the third generation of mice, there was a 50% infant mortality rate, as compared to less than 5% normal mortality rate. The continuous stress response elicited from the experimental animals resulted in increased susceptibility to disease, for it exhausted the defense system. Dr. Becker concluded that in mice or in humans such stress could be expected to result in an increase in such conditions as hypertension and behavioral abnormalities, as well as an increase in degenerative diseases, especially those associated with decreased immune competency such as cancer. He also suggested that, under such stress, previously harmless organisms would begin to produce new maladies such as Legionnaire's Disease and Reyes' Syndrome of that decade.

Since the time of Becker's experiments, the press has given much coverage to the controversial issue of the hazards of high tension lines and the overall effect of 60 cycle current on health. Making the news today are the potential health hazards associated with the use of cell phones. Their use has been linked with visual problems, as well as headaches, ear problems, brain tumors and short term memory loss.[1] "Tests have revealed that a person's brain waves (EEG) are affected by a cell phone used at a distance of up to 300 feet."[2]

Epidemiological studies have shown higher-than-average rates of leukemia and brain cancer among electrical workers and among children residing near high-tension power lines. A University of Colorado study found that the death rate for certain cancers is twice the average for people living within 130 feet of high-voltage power lines. At distances between 100 feet and 2000 feet, the following have been observed: stunted growth, decreased calcium flow, abnormal EEGs, changes in blood chemistry and heart rate and drops in human reaction time. It has also been found that radiation in the ELF range can stimulate the release of stress hormones in chimpanzees, leading to immune suppression.

We live in a virtual sea of electromagnetic pollution with all manner of radiation being emitted from such sources as video display terminals, microwave ovens, hair dryers, electric blankets, beepers, water beds, standard household appliances, televisions, telephones, an array of sophisticated medical diagnostic equipment and more. To gauge the effects of 60 cycle current, hold a switched-on hairdryer in one hand, and have someone muscle test the other arm. In all probability, the muscle will weaken, demonstrating the short circuit created in your body by the incompatible frequency.

Electric blankets and water beds can be especially harmful since we're exposed to their radiations for a prolonged period while sleeping. There has been found to be a higher incidence of miscarriages among women who use electric blankets than among women who do not. Miscarriage rates are also significantly higher (about doubled) among women who spend at least 20 hours per week in front of a video display terminal at their jobs.

Wall outlets leak radiation, and if you have one at the head of your bed, whether turned on or not, 60 cycle current will be beamed at your head, affecting pituitary and pineal function.

Due to the electric (and now electronic) nature of our society, "the average American now gets a daily dose of electromagnetic radiation up to 200 million times more intense than what his ancestors took in from the sun, stars and other natural sources."[3]

W. Ross Adey of the Brain Research Institute of UCLA did an experiment in 1973 where he exposed monkeys to the electrical radiation present in our every day environment. He found that the animals demonstrated changes in behavior and had a distorted sense of time. Adey concluded that exposure to electromagnetic pollution alters our natural biological rhythms. Artificial electromagnetic force fields created by power lines override the earth's natural magnetism, and the body responds by adjusting to the pulse of the artificial signals, thus creating the stress response. The body's internal clock becomes altered due to decreased melatonin production by the pineal gland caused by ELF waves.

Soviet scientists have found that exposure to household appliances can cause central nervous system disorders. In vitro studies have shown that a one gauss field (such as found around household appliances) can significantly inhibit cell growth.

Russia seems to be ahead of the U.S. in their study of the effects of electromagnetic radiation. Their microwave emission standards are *1000 times* stricter than ours (their one *microwatt* per square centimeter vs. our one *milliwatt*). Microwaves are very short waves of electromagnetic energy that travel at the speed of light. Much of our modern technology uses microwaves — radar, beepers, microwave ovens, CB and ham radios, remote phones and diathermy units. The thermal effect of high energy pulsed microwaves is known to be damaging and was the only effect recognized by America when we set our emission standards. Non-thermal dangers have been documented in the U.S., but military and industrial spokesmen have refused to acknowledge them. The Russians, however, have acknowledged numerous adverse effects of microwaves, including headaches, dizziness, eye pain, sleeplessness, irritability, anxiety, stomach pain, nervous tension, inability to concentrate, hair loss, in addition to an increased incidence of appendicitis, cataracts, reproductive problems and cancer.

In 1959, John Heller found that garlic sprouts irradiated with low levels of microwaves showed chromosome damage. Also in that year, a Scarsdale, New York ophthalmologist began a study of the effect of microwave exposure on radar maintenance men for the Air Force. Examining the lens of the eye, he found no abnormalities, but a few years later, he found that microwave workers tended to develop cataracts behind the lens. In 1964, a group of researchers at John Hopkins School of Medicine found a correlation between Downs Syndrome and parental exposure to radar.

One of the most dangerous applications of microwave technology was in the development of the microwave oven. Documented dangers of this device prompted the Russians to ban the use of microwave ovens in 1976. Today, over 90% of American homes use these ovens for meal preparation. When it was first sold, the maximum leakage permitted from the microwave oven was 5 milliwatts per square centimeter — five times the present emissions standards. Many recalls were necessary in order to fix ovens that leaked more than the standard. Research has not established *any* level of radiation to be safe. The effects of low level radiation are insidious because they cannot be felt and are cumulative. It has been established that the nervous system in humans is affected by microwave exposure which is 300 times below established "safety" levels. In view of the evidence, I do not endorse the use of microwave ovens due to the fact that they all leak some amount of radiation. Apart from the dangers posed by radiation leakage, there appear also to be health hazards posed by the consumption of microwave-heated foods. In 1991, a Swiss scientist, Hans Ulrich Hertel, co-published a research paper indicating that food cooked in microwave ovens caused significant changes in the blood of those who ate it. These changes included a decrease in hemoglobin, cholesterol values and lymphocyte count. All such changes were abnormal, of a degenerative nature.

Hertel was prevented from making his findings known to the public, for the Swiss Association of Dealers for Electroapparatuses for Households and Industry had a "gag order" issued to silence him. Happily, that order was recinded in 1998 by the European Court of Human Rights.(4) In the same year that Hertel was publishing his findings on microwave ovens (1991), there was a lawsuit in Oklahoma concerning the hospital use of a microwave oven to warm blood for a transfusion. A patient had died from the microwave-heated blood transfusion.

It is a little-known fact that microwave ovens were invented by the Nazis for use in their mobile support operations during their invasion of Russia. Russian, German and Swiss research point to many health problems resulting from the continual ingestion of microwaved foods. Long-term results include:

1) Permanent brain damage caused by "shorting out" of electrical impulses in the brain.
2) Inability of the body to metabolize the unknown by-products created in microwaved food.
3) Alteration or shut down of both male and female hormone production.
4) Reduction or alteration of minerals, vitamins and other nutrients.
5) Alteration of minerals in vegetables into cancerous free radicals.
6) Stomach and intestinal cancerous growths (tumors).
7) Increase in cancerous cells in human blood.
8) Immune system deficiencies through lymph gland and blood serum alterations.
9) Loss of memory, concentration, emotional stability and a decrease of intelligence.

(This information comes from http://Lawgiver.org)

In 1962, our CIA found that the Soviets were beaming radar-like microwaves into the American Embassy in Moscow. Although the intensity of the radiation was only .002 of the level considered dangerous by American guidelines, significant health impairments resulted. Blood tests of embassy personnel revealed that 1/3 had white blood cell counts almost 50% higher than normal, a sign of severe infection, also present in leukemia. A greater than chance number of appendectomies were performed on embassy personnel who resided on the sixth floor where the energy was the greatest.

It seems that microwave energy attacks the hollow parts of the body (appendix, eyes, genitals) because reduced blood supply there makes these organs more susceptible to microwave thermal effects. The U.S. State Department did not take steps to shield the embassy from the microwave transmissions for another 14 years. By 1980, two U.S. ambassadors present in Moscow at the time of the transmissions had died of cancer. The remaining personnel exhibited a higher than average rate of cancer.

The Navy has experimented with ELF transmitters for "communication purposes" resulting in the development of adverse symptoms in some of their technicians. Those symptoms included high levels of serum triglycerides, as well as a decline in the ability of some of the men to perform simple addition. For these reasons, the Navy abandoned operating the ELF transmitters we were told in a January 1980 issue of *Readers Digest.* Dr. Andrija Puharich, M.D., LL.D., tells us otherwise. He speaks of other applications our military and others have made of ELF transmissions.

Dr. Puharich is a foremost authority on ELF. In addition to being a medical doctor and a lawyer, he is a physicist and inventor with over 75 patents in medical technology. He has also done extensive research in the field of ESP. Dr. Puharich claims that, beginning with Soviet transmissions on 7/4/76, many countries (including ours) have been engaged in ELF warfare, transmitting damaging frequencies to their enemies. These harmful ELF frequencies penetrate the body and influence cellular change at the DNA level, according to Dr. Puharich. They penetrate all barriers without losing their momentum, being stopped only by the DNA. Because it interacts with the DNA molecule, ELF can literally "turn on" or "turn off" any gene, once the correct frequency is known. Specific frequencies have specific effects: One frequency can create a certain kind of cancer in rats in two days; another can reverse it. A certain frequency can turn off the insulin producing mechanism in the pancreas. Depression, anxiety and even mob behavior can be induced by specific frequencies, and this can be accomplished from the other side of the globe!

Dr. Puharich tells us that our military has conducted secret tests on ELF and has transmitted the frequencies, keeping the information classified. He claims that the CIA has attempted to prevent him from speaking out on the dangers of ELF. They have not been successful.

Dr. Robert 0. Becker describes the first Russian signal, broadcast during the U.S. bicentennial celebration, as lying between 3.26 and 17.54 megahertz — a pulsed modulation of a high frequency radio signal. This would place it technically above the ELF range. The signal became known as the "woodpecker" because of the tapping sounds it made. It was so strong originally that it interfered with several communications channels. Within a couple of years after woodpecker began transmitting, persistent physical complaints of mysterious symptoms began to be reported from people in several U.S. cities and Canada. The complaints seemed to be concentrated in Eugene, Oregon. The exact purpose of woodpecker is unknown. Becker, however, concluded that "the available evidence seems to suggest that the Russian woodpecker is a multi-purpose radiation that combines a submarine link with an experimental attack on the American people. It may be intended to increase cancer rates, interfere with decision-making ability, and/or sow confusion and irritation. It may be succeeding."[5]

In 5/90, the EPA released preliminary information about a draft report prepared by its Office of Health and Environmental Assessment that acknowledges a link between cancer and ELF fields. The director, William McFarland, stated, however, that the evidence showed only a *statistical* and not a causal link. What he did not reveal was that his own staff had recommended in the initial draft report that ELF fields be classified as "probable human carcinogens" and that this classification, which would have mandated measures to protect the public health, was deleted from the executive summary of the EPA report after a meeting on 3/6/90 between agency officials and the White House Office of Policy Development.[6]   The public therefore is on its own to uncover information found but not revealed by the government.

It should be noted that not all ELF frequencies are harmful. Many of the physiological effects which are inhibited by one frequency can be enhanced by another. Certain diseases can be cured by altering the frequency (remember the work of Royal Rife?), and the aging process of cells can actually be slowed down. Non-invasive genetic engineering can be accomplished through the manipulation of frequency.

Dan Carlson's application of high frequency sound to accelerate plant growth is an example of a creative and beneficial use of frequency. Carlson obtained the Guiness World Record for an indoor plant by growing a purple passion plant, normally 18" high, to a length of 800 feet! Application of his techniques has produced 20 foot corn stalks, 15 foot tomato plants, as well as huge potatoes, beans, collards, cabbages, etc. Carlson has developed a product that he calls "Sonic Bloom." Sonic Bloom techniques consist of the use of a specific sound frequency around the 5 kilohertz range (identical to bird song) imbedded in Indian sitar music, followed by the application of a special nutrient solution to the plants. The frequency seems to open them up to maximum assimilation of the nutrients. (Order Sonic Bloom home kits from http://www.earthpulse.com/products/sonic.html or voice mail: 907-249-9111.)

The most beneficial ELF frequencies, Dr. Puharich found, fall in the 7-9 Hertz range. 7.83 Hertz is the natural resonant frequency of our planet. This approximate 8 Hertz frequency therefore has a healing effect. So, too, does any harmonic (or multiple) of 8. This may mean that, had we built our electrical grid system on 64 cycles per second rather than 60, we would be in a lot better shape than we are now! Dr. Puharich tells us that the hands of the psychic or spiritual healer emit a constant 8 Hertz frequency. To counteract the detrimental effects of ELF, Dr. Puharich developed one of the first personal "shielding devices" on the market. As public awareness grows regarding electromagnetic pollution, more and more such devices have been developed. Many of them broadcast the earth's natural resonant frequency, the 7.83 hertz. Several companies are now also producing shields for video display terminal (VDT) screens. While acrylic and lead materials screen out UV and x-rays, they do not combat the microwave emissions emanating from VDT screens, nor the ELF and VLF (very low frequency) emitted by the transformers. Televisions, as well as computers, radiate these frequencies. Items for detecting electromagnetic disturbances and shielding both the body and the indoor environment from them are available through The Cutting Edge Catalog (www.cutcat.com, 800-497-9516). Where computers are concerned, use of a laptop model is a safe alternative, for the screen does not emit harmful radiations.

In consideration of ELF warfare, as well as our use of 60 cycle current, microwave technology and all the other sources of electromagnetic radiation currently affecting our planet, some form of shielding device may well be an indispensable item of personal protection for informed individuals. It is also the better part of wisdom to avoid living near power lines and transmitting towers and to keep household appliances to a minimum (an electric toothbrush is not a necessity!). Additionally, it is advisable to assure an adequate intake of the antioxidant nutrients (discussed earlier), which provide protection against the effects of ionizing radiation. These are best obtained from whole foods.

AN EXPERT SPEAKS

I was delighted to learn many years ago that a friend, Will Spates, had started his own indoor environmental inspection business. I had met Will just before leaving Tampa in 1993 when he was introduced to me by Helmut Ziehe, the man who brought Baubiologie (building biology) to the U.S. from Germany. Helmut founded the Clearwater Baubiologie Institute. Will trained in Europe with Wolfgang Maes and also studied with Reinhard Fuchs, director of the Baubiologie and Ecology Institute of New Zealand. He has worked with and taught at the Clearwater Baubiologie Institute.

After hearing about Indoor Environmental Technologies, Will's company, I contacted him and subsequently had my home inspected. What a learning experience! — one that renewed my interest in the factors leading to environmental illness. These include, but are not limited to, electromagnetic pollution. My association with Will subsequently gave birth to a jointly authored article that appeared in the October 1995 edition of the *Sarasota Eco*. What follows is a reproduction of the original draft of that article:

INSIDE ENVIRONMENTAL ILLNESS

The World Health Organization reports that 90% of chronic illness is related to environmental factors. We tend to think of pollution as an outdoor problem, but the fact of the matter is that the average indoor environment is <u>more</u> polluted, containing hazardous chemicals in concentrations 10 to 40 times greater than those found outside. The EPA estimates that 11,400 people were killed last year from indoor pollution. Some contaminants can be more dangerous indoors than out due to lack of adequate ventilation, especially in homes/offices sealed up to conserve energy. Considering the fact that the average person spends 90% of his time indoors, he is at significant risk for developing environmental illness. This risk can be minimized, however, by identifying and removing or reducing indoor pollutants. The first step toward solving the problem is to become aware of its existance.

Allergies

Environmental illness is triggered by maladaptive responses to virtually anything in our environment — chemicals, foods, inhalants, electromagnetic radiation. It can result from the toxic effect of pollutants or from an allergic reaction to non-toxic substances. We're all familiar with sneezy, runny-nose type allergic responses. Less well-known are what William Philpott, M.D., refers to as *Brain Allergies* (book by that title published in 1980). He and other prominent medical doctors (including Sherry Rogers, author of *Tired or Toxic)* present us with convincing evidence that virtually any disorder — physical, mental or emotional — can result from allergic responses.

Such concepts as "cereal grain psychoses" or "hydrocarbon- induced suicidal ideation" are foreign to most and will take time to filter into mainstream thinking. The emerging field of "clinical ecology" concerns itself with such atypical allergies. The first step in solving the problem involves identifying the allergen (allergy-inducing substance). Efforts will then be focused on "desensitizing" the subject, usually by limiting (and sometimes cycling) exposure to the allergen and upgrading nutritional status. A promising new technique, Nambudripad Allergy Elimination Technique (NAET), involves combining Applied Kinesiology (muscle-testing) and acupuncture techniques to reprogram the body and eliminate the maladaptive response.

When a maladaptive response is not serving the best interests of the body, it is desirable to eliminate that response whenever possible. There are instances, however, when such responses do serve us in that they warn of the toxicity of the offending substance or pollutant. In this case, in addition to strengthening the body, steps must be taken to eliminate or minimize the harmful effects of the pollutant by removing it or altering it in some way.

Sick Building Syndrome

Most indoor environments are loaded with pollutants. They can be chemical and/or electromagnetic in nature. Chemical pollutants can be found in air and water supplies and in many building materials and household items. Studies show that your risk of getting cancer from exposure to chemicals in the water and air in your home is greater than your risk from exposure to the same chemicals in a hazardous waste site!

Electromagnetic pollution comes to us in the form of alternating electrical fields, alternating magnetic fields, electrical direct fields, magnetic direct fields and earth radiations. These fields can be generated from such unlikely sources as mobile phones, synthetic carpets, stuffed animals, spring mattresses, "geopathic" zones, fluorescent lamps, computer terminals and wallpaper. For reasons not entirely understood, allergic responses have often been eliminated when these fields are reduced, minimizing or eliminating electromagnetic stressors.

Illness resulting from stress factors in the indoor environment is known as "Sick Building Syndrome." It affects an estimated 40 million Americans. Most doctors are not trained to recognize this syndrome and will therefore only treat the patient's symptoms, which of course will never be eliminated until the cause is discovered and removed. If you suffer from a condition of unknown etiology, it may benefit you tremendously to have your home and/or office inspected by someone trained in "Baubiologie." This science of building biology comes to us from Germany where it is widely respected and practiced. Those trained in it are capable of identifying and rectifying stress factors in indoor environments. The result is often a pronounced improvement in the health of those who live or work in the formerly "sick" building.

Electromagnetic Pollution

According to Wolgang Maes, father of Baubiologie inspections, "No other single artificial factor has stranger offshoots than (the) electrification of our living space." This "electrification" — from radio and TV transmitters, radar installations, radio and TV relay systems, microwave units and earth satellites — has completely obscured the normal level of natural earth radiation.

Interestingly, the dominant brain wave frequency for all life on earth is 10 hertz (or cycles per second). This corresponds to the natural rhythm of the earth. Ten hertz brain wave patterns are indicative of a relaxed "alpha" state. When the mind is active, beta waves up to 30 hertz are produced. Our entire electrical grid system, however, doubles that frequency, running on 60 cycle current. Engulfed in a maze of electromagnetic radiation, the body of modern man is therefore under constant biological stress. It has been established through the pioneering work of Robert O. Becker, M.D., that such stressful conditions significantly impair immunity and set the stage for development of degenerative disease.

Animal studies link electromagnetic fields to changes in blood chemistry, cell growth, brain function and hormone production, and implicate them in tumor development and growth, miscarriage and birth defects. A study of 1600 pregnancies conducted by Kaiser Permanente in California revealed that women who spent more than 20 hours per week in front of a computer video display terminal had 73% more miscarriages than women who did not have such exposure.

Electromagnetic fields can also suppress the pineal gland's secretion of the regulating hormone melatonin, resulting in depression, mood changes and psychiatric disorders. Melatonin inhibits tumor growth by increasing the cytotoxicity of the lymphocytes, the body's natural killer cells. Suppression of its production by the pineal gland has been linked to development of melanoma and cancers of the breast, ovaries and prostate. Secretions from the pineal gland are synchronized with the earth's resonant frequency, between 7 and 10 hertz. It is through the antenna of this gland that we are tied to the energy of the earth.

Clinical studies have shown that the following reactions have resulted from exposure to "modest" electromagnetic fields in the home or workplace: fatigue, migraines, cramps, pain in the glands, speech impediments, shortness of breath, unconsciousness and allergies. Noticeable changes in heart activity have also been observed. It has additionally been demonstrated that women using electric heating pads during pregnancy had significantly more premature births.

Electrical Alternating Fields

Electrical alternating fields come from electrical alternating voltage — 110 volts with a 60 hertz frequency in the U.S. and 220 volts with 50 hertz in Europe. Radiations are emitted from all junction boxes, sockets, cables and devices with main connections — *even when there is no current.*

Faulty house wiring and defective or non-existent grounding can greatly amplify the electrical fields produced from these sources. So too can the use of too many cables and electrical devices in close proximity to the body.

The Baubiologie inspector measures alternating fields with a voltmeter. Measurements are taken from walls, cables, sockets — and the human body. The body measurement is typically taken with the subject lying in his bed, for a good 8 hours per night is usually spent in this location, and during the passive state of sleep, the body is 10-100 times more vulnerable to electrical stimuli. Ideally, the voltmeter would register zero, although a measurement up to 20 millivolts is tolerable. However, studies have shown that even measurements as low as 15-20 millivolts can cause nerve stress.

Amazingly, body measurements in the *thousands* and even *hundreds of thousands* of millivolts have been recorded. Here are some examples from the files of Wolfgang Maes:

CASE #1
MEASUREMENT: **4,500** millivolts
SYMPTOMS: Bedwetting from age 5 (subject 13 years of age), hay fever, allergy to dust mites
SOLUTION: Install "cut-off switch" at fuse box to combat faulty electrical installation in the wall

CASE #2
MEASUREMENT: **6,000** millivolts
SYMPTOMS: Stress, strain, insomnia, back pain
SOLUTION: Switching off the cable running to the bedroom at the fuse box to remove strong fields coming from the wall

CASE #3
MEASUREMENT: **35,000** millivolts
SYMPTOMS: Severe back pain, migraines, dizziness, heart attacks
SOLUTION: Removal of electric bed, electric heating pad; repair of defects in cable of bedroom wall

CASE #4
MEASUREMENT: **155,000** millivolts
SYMPTOMS: Heart attacks, circulation disruption, "mysterious & intolerable pain" (ambulance came every other night; subject 40 years old)
SOLUTION: Repair of faulty electrical heating unit of water bed

In all of the above cases, the subjects became symptom-free once steps were taken to reduce the electrical fields in their bedrooms. There are actions we can take to minimize electrical fields in our homes, especially in the sleeping area. As mentioned above, electrical defects can be repaired, power shut off at the fuse box, or a cutoff switch can be installed in the fuse box. We can also reduce fields by simply unplugging electrical appliances at night.

Alternating Magnetic Fields

Magnetic fields are generated from current-consuming devices that are switched on and remain in operation. These alternating fields will penetrate solid matter — building materials, walls, ceilings and the human body — without being absorbed by it.

Epidemiological studies have repeatedly shown that children who live near high tension lines and electrical workers have a significantly increased incidence of leukemia and brain cancer. The press has made us aware of the potential hazards of residing near high tension lines. What most of us are not aware of is that many devices in our homes and offices actually produce the same high magnitude fields as those generated by high tension lines.

To avoid the harmful effects of alternating magnetic fields, it is necessary to either turn off the radiating device or to maintain a safe distance from it. Items with particularly strong fields include fuse boxes, fluorescent and halogen lamps, TVs and electrical alarm clocks. Maintaining a distance of 2-3 yards from these items is usually sufficient to avoid harm from their fields. The radiation from incandescent bulbs is minimal and they are therefore to be preferred over conventional fluorescents. Full-spectrum lights are recommended over standard ones — these provide the best quality light and are available in fluorescent tubes and bulbs.

Under floor electrical heating systems also radiate strong alternating magnetic fields and should not be used, especially in the bedroom. Small, low-volt lamps can be a hazard as well, as their transformers produce large magnetic fields. Any items requiring transformers to operate should be avoided, for the transformers often consume current and radiate fields even when switched off. Beware of devices that have built-in transformers.

Both electrical and magnetic alternating fields produce current in the human body. Magnetic field strength can be measured in units known as Tesla (T). The ideal measurement of zero nanotesla (a billionth part Tesla) is rarely found today. A typical downtown area measures 20-50 nanotesla. Bedroom measurements should ideally not exceed 20 nanotesla, and under no circumstances should they ever exceed 100. Here again are some cases from the files of Wolfgang Maes:

CASE #1

MEASUREMENT:	**3,000 Nanotesla** (measured at the workplace of the subject)
SYMPTOM:	"Terrible headaches"
SOURCE:	A slide projector used by the subject (He typically stood a few inches from it)
SOLUTION:	Subject moved more than a yard away from the projector, operating it by remote control

CASE #2

MEASUREMENT:	**600 Nanotesla** (measured in the crib of a baby)
SYMPTOM:	Screaming attacks every night
SOURCE:	Baby phone (remote listening device) installed in crib about 8" from the baby
SOLUTION:	Removal of baby phone

Wolfgang Maes himself recovered from diabetes and heart, circulation and digestive problems after removing all electromagnetic fields from his bedroom. His experience drove him to switch professions (from journalism to Baubiologie) so he could share his information with others. He now does home inspections on physician referral in his native Germany.

Electric Direct Fields

Electrical fields can be produced in the absence of voltage. They are without frequency. Synthetic products and plastic materials can produce these static fields, often referred to as "electrostatic charges." These electrostatic charges can be emitted from carpets, wallpaper, furniture, lacquers, plastic foils and bags, foamed plastics, garments, computer screens, television sets and terminals. Electrostatic charges also occur from natural materials such as silk and wool. These discharge very quickly, however, in comparison to plastics, which discharge slowly, if at all. Moreover, the charges from nature have a positive field or polarization, while those from artificial elements are often negative, with unnaturally high potentials.

As Maes points out, walking on synthetic carpets with plastic soled shoes generates an "enormous artificial electrical power in our bodies." Electrostatic charges increase with friction and dry air. Electrostatically charged synthetic materials also disrupt the ionization of the air, adversely affecting its quality and creating a build-up of tension in the body. Allergic and asthmatic people are particularly sensitive to changes in the climate of rooms from electrostatic loads, as the artificial loading and depolarization of the air can cause allergy-producing particles to increase a thousand fold. Natural air produces an electrostatic balance of about 100-200 volts per meter (V/m), while loaded rooms can yield readings as high as 1,000-30,000 V/m.

Synthetic carpets can produce the same magnitude of fields as those produced by television and computer screens. Children who crawl around on these floors suffer most. They are also adversely affected by stuffed animal toys made from strongly radiating synthetics. These cuddly toys can produce an electrostatic field measuring as high as 80,000 V/m.

To minimize electric direct fields in the home, it is advisable to ground all conducting materials, increase air humidity, cover synthetic materials with natural ones, remove all metal screens from bedrooms (they produce high voltages and remain loaded for hours or even days), avoid the use of plastics and synthetics wherever possible, and use only natural wallpapers, floor and bed coverings.

Magnetic Direct Fields

Artificial magnetic fields can penetrate the sleeping body via beds made with or surrounded by steel. The magnetic disturbance is reflected in variations of compass readings when the device is slowly moved from head to foot of the bed. Spring mattresses, steel beds, frames for spring mattresses, hinges on the headboards, metal items stored underneath the bed — all can create magnetic disturbance. In the work place, the common office chair is a source of large magnetic fields that can adversely affect the abdominal organs. Researchers and medical experts see a close connection between permanent magnetic fields and corresponding local disease. These fields have been linked to cancer, birth defects, still births, heart attacks, circulatory disturbances, muscle cramps and metabolic disorders.

Magnetic fields cannot be demagnetized. The only solution is to remove the offending metal. It is especially important to keep your bed absolutely free of metal — and remember that magnetic fields can penetrate walls. For this reason, it is not wise to sleep in bedrooms above garages: Cars parked below produce large magnetic fields. In placement of your bed, stay at least a yard away from door frames and at least 16" above the floor.

Earth Radiation

Underground water veins and earth dislocations are sources of intensified earth radiations. The distortion of terrestrial magnetic fields is measurable on the surface of the earth above the geological disturbance, but its application to rooms does not appear to be reliable. Measurement of these radiations can be problematic. What seems to be significant is the fact that rises in natural radioactivity can be detected above geological disturbances. Values of 100% or more are reflected on radiometers if the measurement is above a geopathic zone. There does appear to be a relationship between subterranean water sources and ionizing radioactive radiation. Where beds are placed exactly above geopathic zones, higher incidences of cancer are recorded.

Maes states that he has found houses where the radioactive radiation was higher than that resulting from the Chernobyl incident. The source of such radiation was not geological disturbance, however — it was radioactive construction materials: cinders, ashes, chemical gypsum, tiles, pumice and metallurgical stones. He sites several cases of brain tumors where radioactivity coming from these items was several times higher than the law allows for workers in nuclear power plants.

Chemicals

Up to 80% of the materials used in any indoor environment are artificial. Outgassing of dangerous chemicals from these artificial materials has been associated with building-related illness.

Materials to avoid in the home and work place are wall to wall plastic carpets and foam carpet pads, paints with Volatile Organic Compounds (VOCs) and mildewcides, synthetic materials, plywood and particle board. Moisture-damaged building materials (as well as high humidity and condensation) also pose a problem in that they create an environment that supports the rapid and continuous growth of molds, mildews and bacteria. Exposure to these microbiological and chemical contaminants can result in such allergy-like symptoms as eye, nose and throat irritation, headache, fatigue and dizziness. Chronic exposure can lead to hypersensitivity pneumonitis, allergic asthma and chronic allergy symptoms. Research indicates that there has been a five-fold increase in asthma in children in the last 20 years.

Over 3 dozen chemicals may be found in synthetic carpets. Among the hazardous chemicals outgassed by carpets (for up to 5 years after installation) are formaldehyde, xylene and ethylbenzene. Carpets over 5 years old usually have stopped outgassing. However, they then become a breeding ground for dust mites and mold.

Volatile Organic Compounds

The adhesives used for carpets contain VOCs. VOCs are chemically unstable compounds that vaporize (turn to gas) readily. They may combine with other chemicals to create compounds that can cause toxic reactions when inhaled or absorbed through the skin. Many VOCs are suspected carcinogens. Known side effects include eye and respiratory tract irritation, headaches, dizziness, visual distortions, impaired memory, depression, kidney problems, migraines, wheezing, asthma and nervous system damage. VOCs are found in paints, varnishes and wax. Other products that can release them include stored fuels, products used for cleaning, disinfecting and degreasing; cosmetics, moth repellents, air fresheners and aerosol sprays.

Formaldehyde

Synthetic carpets are just one of many formaldehyde-containing items found in the indoor environment. Particle board is made from wood shavings that are saturated with urea-formaldehyde resin and then pressed into wood-like form. Plywood consists of several sheets of wood pressed together with phenol-formaldehyde resin. Formaldehyde is emitted by many construction materials and household products that contain formaldehyde-based glues, resins, preservatives and bonding agents. It is also found in smoke and unvented fuel-burning appliances and in paper goods, household cleaners and foam insulation.

Many textile products, including nylon, all polyester/cotton blends and permanent press fabrics, have formaldehyde finishes. Formaldehyde exposure can cause burning, watery eyes, nausea, burning throat, skin rash, cough, tiredness, excessive thirst, nosebleeds, insomnia, difficult breathing and disorientation. High concentrations can trigger asthma attacks. Formaldehyde is a known carcinogen in animals and a suspected one in humans. Potted plants, such as aloe, spider and corn plants, can help absorb formaldehyde. Use 1-2 potted plants per 100 square feet.

A home inspection will reveal any of the above problems you may have in your indoor environment. For information on home or office inspections, you may contact Will Spates at 727-446-7717 in Clearwater, FL. He does both home and office inspections, mostly in Florida. Will has, on occasion, traveled outside the state (and even outside of the country) to do inspections. If he's unable to come to you, he can connect you with someone qualified in your area who can do the inspection. Visit his web site at www.iet.baweb.com. Contact the Baubiologie Institute (727-461-4371) for information on their seminars and Environmental Inspector & Consultant training, or check out their website at: www.bau-biologieusa.com.

As time passes and environmental illness increases, I predict we'll see an upsurge in businesses such as Indoor Environmental Technologies. There is certainly a great need for them in order to identify and rectify the problems of electromagnetic pollution and other types of pollution found in indoor environments.

CHAPTER 9

Essential Nutrients (Macronutrients)

"Supplements are the ultimate fast food."
Paul Bergner

There are six "essential" nutrients: protein, fats, carbohydrates, vitamins, minerals and water. The first three of these are known as "macronutrients," as they're needed in large amounts by the body. It is these macronutrients that will be discussed in this chapter. All foods are composed of all of them to one degree or another; generally one or another predominates, however.

PROTEIN

The foods highest in protein are meat, dairy products, nuts, seeds and legumes. This means they are composed primarily of protein. While protein is an essential nutrient, without which we could not exist, unless it is broken down into its constituent amino acids, it is useless and toxic to the body. The intake of large amounts of protein is by no means assurance that the body will be able to break it down into amino acids. In fact, over-consumption of protein causes many undesirable conditions including kidney damage, osteoporosis, arthritis, atherosclerosis, immune deficiency and has been linked to breast, liver and bladder cancer, as well as to leukemia. Let's take a look at the link between high protein intake and disease formation.

As you're aware from information previously presented, most of our high protein foods are acid-forming in the system. When the body becomes too acid, toxic build-up occurs, for toxins are of an acid nature. When there is an acid build-up, the system retains water to neutralize it, as in Dr. West's "trapped plasma protein" model. Over-consumption of meat and other high protein foods causes a depletion of our alkaline reserves, forcing the body to withdraw alkaline minerals from its own tissues to buffer excess acid.

Excessive consumption of protein also causes over-stimulation of the pancreas, resulting in reduced enzyme activity. Since enzymes are needed to break foods down into their constituent parts for digestion, the result is poor digestion of proteins into amino acids. Protein then becomes a poison to the body, which has difficulty producing adequate enzymes, hormones, antibodies and new tissue. Excessive demands are therefore made on vitamins and minerals (especially B6, zinc and magnesium), leading to nutrient deficiencies. The net result is impaired immunity, which can lead to all manner of disease.

Abundant stomach acid is essential for proper digestion of protein. Carnivores have stomach acid that is twenty times stronger than that of humans, well equipping them to handle large quantities of meat. The human is more of an omnivore by design.

Meat is a food that contains no fiber and is low in water content. Therefore, it tends to clog the colon, adversely affecting elimination, if not consumed in concert with high-fiber foods such as vegetables. Over-consumption of meat can also lead to a calcium/phosphorous imbalance, with too much phosphorous leading to calcium deficiency.

Protein requirements are not the same for all of us. They vary according to the nutritional status, body size and activity of the individual. Differences in metabolic rate (fast or slow oxidation, or conversion of food to energy), ancestry (did our ancestors come from a cold or warm climate?) and blood type also have an impact on an individual's protein needs. Most blood types don't do well on a strict vegetarian diet.

I do believe this: A vegetarian diet is indicated for people when they are ill, for it helps to readily rebuild the alkaline reserve and provides an abundance of bioavailable vitamins and minerals. Once health is rebuilt, however, many people will decompensate without animal products in their diet. Just a little egg yolk and raw cheese will do nicely if you're averse to eating animal flesh. It takes extensive knowledge of nutrition (and the right body type) to be a successful vegan, however. Without the liberal incorporation of a variety of nuts and seeds, fermented soybean products (unfermented ones are indigestible) and sea vegetables, the vegan will likely over-consume carbohydrates in the form of grains and in so doing, open the door to a host of health problems.

The National Research Council recommends the daily consumption of 0.42 grams of protein per pound of body weight. That would be an intake of 75 grams for an individual weighing 150 pounds. This is basically the same recommendation that nutrition pioneer, Adelle Davis, was making in the 1960s: consumption of ½ gram of protein per pound of body weight. An intake of far less protein — 25-50 grams per day — appears to be optimal for most people, however. Beyond that amount, we are subject to development of the conditions described above, as well as declining strength and endurance.

The average American on the SAD takes in a great deal more protein than is recommended. An intake of between 90 and 100 grams daily is not uncommon. This is unequivocally excessive. It has been found that consumption of more than 6 oz. of animal protein *cuts oxygen intake by 60%.*(1)   Oxygen, you will recall, is essential to ATP production and therefore to creation of energy at the cellular level. Also, cancer cells thrive where oxygen is under-supplied.

The average American eats 150 pounds of pork, beef and other red meat per year. We would be well advised to reduce our consumption. Meat is a highly stimulatory food, however, and to give it up all at once and totally could be devastating for the person used to taking in large amounts. It is best therefore to slowly and gradually reduce the amount of meat consumed to give the body a chance to adapt. Also, I believe it is vitally important to avoid commercial meats, laced as they are with antibiotics and steroids, as well as the imprinted misery of the diseased factory-farm animal who lived a life deprived of healthful conditions. Select organic meats. These come from animals that were well nourished and not drugged.

While I have cautioned against the ill effects of excessive protein consumption, let me balance that out by stressing the importance of including an adequate amount of good quality protein in the diet. Protein is vitally important for tissue growth and repair and numerous bodily functions. However, protein utilization is problematic for most of us. Despite the large number of grams of protein consumed daily by the majority of Americans, protein deficiency is not uncommon, due to the body's inability to properly utilize it. Also, the over-consumption of carbohydrates creates a low protein to carbohydrate ratio, resulting in a *relative* protein deficiency. This, in turn, leads to hormonal imbalance and subsequently to conditions of overweight and disease. The answer is clearly to reduce the carbs rather than increase the already excessive protein.

The non-essential amino acids (those which the body can produce) are manufactured in the liver *if it is working properly*. Once the body has digested food proteins into amino acids, the liver re-forms them into usable protein structures known as nucleo proteins. This process is called "humanizing" of proteins. Here is where most of us have a problem, with nucleo protein deficiency.

There are many factors that can cause this deficiency. Among them are the consumption of either too little or too much protein and the consumption of "high stress proteins." High stress proteins are those that take more energy than they give. They include pork, lamb, veal, beef, most raw nuts, unfermented soy products, cow's milk, sardines and brewer's yeast (except in small amounts). When proteins and starchy carbohydrates are eaten at the same meal, both cannot be digested, and the body opts to digest the carbs, leaving the protein to putrefy. Proper protein digestion is also inhibited by negative emotions, drinking too much fluid with meals, eating too much food and not getting sufficient exercise (needed to move proteins into the cells).

The SAD is notoriously lacking in vegetables. This is unfortunate because the consumption of vegetables with protein is necessary to provide the "enzymes, assimilation factors, chlorophyll and fiber" to properly utilize that protein.(2) The minerals in the vegetables buffer the pH. They, along with their enzymes, help digest and assimilate the protein.

Stuart Wheelwright's *Pro Vita Plan,* which I have personally followed for several years, is designed to optimize protein digestion and utilization by emphasizing low stress proteins, eaten before 2 p.m., apart from starchy carbohydrates. In the context of this plan, breakfast becomes the major protein meal (albeit, not a bacon, egg and toast breakfast!). There are four major reasons for eating protein early in the day: The body is swinging into an acid pH (needed for protein digestion) at this time, digestive enzymes are at their strongest, and energy flow through the stomach is peaked between 1 and 9 a.m. Digestion and assimilation are therefore optimal at this time. Lastly, proteins tend to have a stimulatory effect, making us alert to face the day (while carbohydrates have a sedative effect and are therefore most properly eaten for the evening meal before we retire).

In the context of the Pro Vita plan, an intake of 22-30 grams of protein per 100# of body weight is recommended. The plan is designed to get maximum use from minimal protein intake, thus avoiding the potential toxicity problems associated with high protein intake.

The *Pro Vita Plan* is built on a foundation of vegetables, while most eating plans are built on a base of grains (starchy carbohydrates). Vegetables are technically carbohydrates also, but Wheelwright makes a distinction between them and other carbohydrates. *The Pro Vita Plan* calls for 5 vegetables; 4 raw and 1 lightly cooked, to be eaten at breakfast and lunch (and also dinner if desired). The raw vegetables provide enzymes that help digest proteins. They also provide the alkaline minerals needed to buffer the acidity of the protein. Starchy vegetables are considered carbohydrates and therefore should not be eaten with proteins. They include boiled beans, potatoes, Jerusalem artichokes, pumpkin, rutabagas, split peas and yams.

The *Pro Vita Plan* also calls for 5 proteins; 4 raw and 1 cooked, to be eaten with the first two meals of the day. The 4 raw proteins can include sprouts, as well as seeds and nuts that have been soaked overnight in water. Dinner should be the lightest meal of the day. This is the time to consume the starchy carbs. Combining them with vegetables is fine — No protein with this meal, however. An option would be to consume a fruit meal for supper. Fruit should not be combined with other foods but rather eaten alone so that it is digested without interference.

For details on the *Pro Vita Plan* and sample menus, read Jack Tip's fine book of the same name available through Apple-A-Day Press (512-328-3996).

ENZYMES

Enzymes are complex proteins that serve as catalysts for nearly every biochemical process in the body. It is their job to structure protein, vitamins and minerals into blood, organs and tissue. Enzymes are found in plant and animal cells and act as organic catalysts in numerous chemical reactions. Their role as catalyst is well known. However, Dr. Edward Howell, biochemist and pioneer in the study of enzymes, who has studied them since 1932, maintains that they are more than mere catalysts, for catalysts are inert substances. Enzymes are not inert; they radiate life energy.

Although so small as to be invisible, even with the most powerful microscopes, enzymes are the basis of all metabolic activity. They facilitate more than 150,000 biochemical reactions and empower every cell in every tissue, gland and organ of the body to function. Enzymes are responsible for the oxidation process in the body. They are a major factor in such processes as growth, metabolism, digestion and cellular reproduction. More and more enzymes are being identified. So far, scientists have identified over 80,000 different enzyme systems.

Enzymes help extract chelated minerals from food and aid in

breaking protein down into amino acids. Without them, we could not breathe, see, digest food or move around. It is enzyme activity that causes food to ripen and spoil and beer to ferment.

There are three classes of enzymes: **metabolic, digestive** and **food** enzymes. It is the metabolic enzymes that run our bodies. They do the structuring of proteins, fats and carbohydrates and are responsible for the repair of tissue damage in the healing process. Our health depends on an adequate supply of metabolic enzymes. Every organ has its own specific metabolic enzymes to perform specialized functions.

The digestive enzymes digest our food. There are three main classes of digestive enzymes: *proteases* (for protein digestion), *amylases* (for carbohydrate digestion) and *lipases* (for fat digestion). Food enzymes, found in raw foods, start the digestive process in the body and help take the load off the digestive enzymes. In 1943, the Physiological Laboratory of Northwestern University did experiments on rats which resulted in the development of the "Law of Adaptive Secretion of Enzymes." This law states that the organism will manufacture enzymes only in the amount needed for any job. If raw foods are consumed, they will be partially digested by their own food enzymes, and the body therefore will make less concentrated digestive enzymes. This law has been confirmed repeatedly through numerous studies in university laboratories. As the law implies, the body values its enzymes. Dr. Howell maintains that all living organisms have a fixed enzyme potential that diminishes with time. When it is exhausted, life ceases. Our enzyme potential is like a bank account. We can choose to withdraw from it frequently or to save and conserve our precious life-sustaining enzymes. Most of us unknowingly are reckless spenders of enzymes. The ingestion of only cooked food demands lavish enzyme secretions from the digestive organs. When we eat cooked food exclusively, we are not taking in any food enzymes with which to digest it, and so the body is forced to produce large amounts of digestive enzymes, thus enlarging digestive organs, especially the pancreas, according to Dr. Howell.

The digestive process requires more energy than any other bodily process. Due to faulty eating habits, such as poor food combining and over-consumption of proteins, most of us have food in our stomachs all the time. Our energy is therefore tied up in the digestive process continually so that there is very little left for other activity.

With so much digestive activity going on constantly and excessive amounts of digestive enzymes being made continually, the body becomes unable to produce an adequate quantity of metabolic enzymes needed for fighting disease and repairing organs. This depletion of metabolic enzymes, due to the body's excessive demand for digestive enzymes, is cited by Dr. Howell as a probable cause of many chronic degenerative diseases such as cancer, heart disease and diabetes.

The excessive demand for production of digestive enzymes is a consequence of our failure to take in sufficient quantities of raw food, for it is raw food only that supplies the food enzymes whose function it is to take the load off the body's digestive enzymes. Dr. Howell tells us that any heat warm enough to feel uncomfortable to the hand is enough to injure enzymes in food. Enzyme destruction takes place at about 116 degrees. The degree of enzyme destruction is a function of time and temperature. In the SAD, we cook almost everything we consume, or it has already been cooked when we purchase it. Any pasteurized product (milk, juice) has been exposed to temperatures of approximately 145 degrees and therefore is devoid of enzymes needed to help digest it. Pasteurization destroys the life force in enzymes. All processed foods have been exposed to heat by one means or another. Processed food therefore is not only short on vitamins and minerals, it is totally devoid of enzymes.

Many authorities in the field of nutrition recommend that the diet consist of anywhere between 50% and 100% raw food (the healthier we are, the more we can comfortably tolerate), with 70-80% being perhaps the most frequent recommendation. Once again, this is a dietary change that is best worked into gradually, for an abrupt change will produce unpleasant symptoms as a result of the body's cleansing activities that are triggered by the raw foods. Including more raw foods in the diet enables the body to produce less concentrated digestive enzymes. If we all took in more exogenous enzymes (from the outside) in the form of raw foods, the body would not have to waste its enzyme potential on digesting foods. By raising our metabolic enzyme potential through increased intake of raw foods and/or enzyme supplements, we increase the body's ability to repair itself. It is the body's metabolic enzyme potential that is its mechanism for curing disease.

Man is the only animal that lives on an enzyme-poor diet. A classic experiment done by Francis Pottenger, M.D., in 1946 dramatically illustrates the effects of such a diet. Dr. Pottenger took

900 cats and divided them into two groups — One was fed raw meat and milk, the other cooked meat and pasteurized milk. Over a ten year period, he found that each successive generation of cats fed cooked food showed an increase in degenerative diseases and other disorders common to man — arthritis, gastritis, liver atrophy, pyorrhea, loss of teeth and hair, osteoporosis, extreme irritability, kidney and thyroid disease, heart disease and cancer, etc. By the third generation, all of these animals were sterile or congenitally malformed. Dr. Pottenger found that it took four generations to correct naturally the inherited damage caused by eating cooked food. None of the cats to whom he'd fed raw foods developed disease. They reproduced normally and lived to a ripe old age.

Cooked food digests much more slowly than raw food. This requires large amounts of energy. Ingestion of raw food conserves energy that can be redirected to rebuilding and repairing damaged tissue. Life span may be increased by increasing intake of raw foods, for in this manner our enzyme potential is conserved. It is not surprising that rats raised on raw food diets lived 30% longer than those raised on cooked foods.

Uncooked foods raise the microelectric potential throughout the body. The stronger the microelectric tensions, the better the ability of the body to repel toxic substances. All toxins are enzyme inhibitors. According to Georges Lakhovsky, eating cooked food physically destroys the oscillating circuit within the cell.

I recommend adding raw fruits and vegetables to the diet, while slowly reducing intake of the more concentrated cooked foods. It may be that the vital force of the body is too depleted to tolerate raw foods initially. In making the transition from the SAD to the optimal diet, it is imperative to go slowly, always adding before subtracting. Start with vegetables and whole grains. Cook them at first, and then, as your vitality level increases, cook them only slightly, and work your way into the introduction of totally raw foods, including fruit. Fruit should never be cooked. It becomes extremely acid-forming. Many of us are so sick that abrupt transition to raw foods would cause a great deal of irritation to the intestines due to the excessive toxicity that is stirred up.

To retain enzyme activity in nuts and seeds, soak them overnight in purified or distilled water or pineapple juice. The purpose of so doing is to release the "enzyme inhibitors" they contain. Nature supplies these foods with enzyme inhibitors to prevent them from germinating prematurely. It is contact with water (or moist soil) that triggers germination. The germination neutralizes or inactivates the enzyme inhibitors. When we soak our nuts and seeds, we are encouraging germination and freeing up enzymes within the foods. Germinating and sprouting increases the enzyme content of foods six to twenty-fold. Soaking grains will also help make them more digestible.

The squirrels in the wild know instinctively about enzyme activity — They bury their nuts. The contact with the moisture in the soil deactivates enzyme inhibitors through germination. By the time the squirrel digs up his nuts, they are digestible.

Considering the lack of enzymes in the SAD, it is not surprising that we spend over two billion dollars per year on digestive aids. Tagamet and Zantac (prescription drugs for gastrointestinal disorders) are top selling drugs in this country.

FATS

Fats in the diet include oils, butter, margarine and lard. All meats, of course, contain a relatively high percentage of fat, some much more than others. Nuts, too, have a high fat content, as do avocados. Fats are the most concentrated source of energy in the diet.

It is essential that we take in a certain amount of fat, for we cannot maintain health on a fat-free diet. Fats serve many vital functions: They facilitate oxygen transport; they lubricate and insulate muscles and organs, aid in the absorption of the fat-soluble vitamins (A ,D, E, K), nourish the skin, mucous membranes and nerves and help maintain body temperature. While fat is an essential nutrient, too much can cause problems. Nearly 40% of the SAD is composed of fat. This is excessive.

The terms "saturated," "monounsaturated" and "polyunsaturated" refer to the way in which the element hydrogen is carried in the fatty acid molecule, to the type and number of hydrogen bonds in the chemical structure of the fatty acids. No fatty food is wholly saturated or unsaturated, only predominately so. The saturated fats are solid at room temperature. The monounsaturated ones are liquid at room temperature but solid when refrigerated, and the polyunsaturates (composed of Omega-3s and Omega-6s) are always liquid, even when refrigerated. The lists below show which oils and fats fall into which categories:

MONOUNSATURATED FATTY ACIDS
olive oil
almond oil
apricot kernel oil
peanut oil
canola oil
high-oleic safflower oil
high-oleic sunflower oil

POLYUNSATURATED FATTY ACIDS

Omega-6s	Omega-3s
vegetable oils	cold-water fish
legumes	(salmon, mackerel,
all nuts, seeds	sardines, tuna,
most grains	herring and anchovies)
breast milk	wild game
organ meats	flax seeds and flax seed oil
lean meats	canola oil
leafy greens	walnuts
borage	pumpkin seeds
evening primrose oil	chia seeds
gooseberry oil	wheat sprouts
black currant oil	soybeans
	fresh sea vegetables
	leafy greens

SATURATED FATS
all meat fats
dairy products
coconut oil
cocoa butter
palm oil
palm-kernel oil
hydrogenated oil

While saturated fats have been implicated in the development of cardiovascular disease, it would appear that the major culprits in this regard are hydrogenated oils (which are artificially saturated), other refined oils and sugar. There is abundant evidence that the body can tolerate, and, indeed, may require, moderate amounts of naturally saturated fats. While our consumption of animal fats has decreased significantly over the last sixty years, the consumption of refined oils, hydrogenated ones (such as margarine and shortening) and refined sugar have increased dramatically, along with a concurrent rise in heart disease.(3)

Refining of oils removes the lecithin, a natural fat emulsifier also produced in the body. Lecithin contains two B vitamins, choline and inositol, which play an important role in maintaining normal blood cholesterol levels. It was long ago demonstrated that "experimental high blood cholesterol cannot be produced by feeding cholesterol and saturated fats if even a minimal amount of lecithin is included in the diet."(4) Lecithin, then, is essential to cholesterol reduction. It has been established that experimental arteriosclerosis can be prevented by giving choline, inositol and the essential fatty acids. Consumption of refined oils, lacking in lecithin, sets us up, then, for cholesterol problems. Refined oils are also lacking in lipase, the enzyme needed to break down fat, as it is destroyed by the heat used in the refining process.

Refined oils are not easy to identify, in that they are not labeled "refined." The aisles of the supermarkets are filled with refined vegetable oils. If stocked at all, the unrefined ones are generally kept in another section, usually a "specialty" or "health food" section. They may also be found in health food stores. Unrefined oils are labeled. Some may actually say "unrefined." More often however, you'll encounter the terms "cold-pressed" or "cold processed." Beware of the cold-pressed oils, as they may have been *pressed* without the use of heat but have been further processed using heat. You may also find the term "expeller pressed." While this method of expelling the oil is less destructive than the standard refining process, it still does not produce a truly unrefined oil. Read your labels. And examine the oils. If they are light and crystal clear, they are refined.

I recommend the exclusive use of unrefined oils. It is also wise to purchase them in small quantities, and store them in the refrigerator, for oils oxidize or turn rancid very rapidly. Recall that three factors cause oxidation — heat, light and oxygen. As soon as we remove the bottle cap, exposing the oil to air, a certain amount of oxidation takes place. Any time oils are used in cooking, of course, the heat can produce rancidity, as can the heat produced at room temperature during storage. Rancid oil does not necessarily smell bad. The major problem with consumption of rancid oil, as previously mentioned, is that it gives rise to free radicals, which, in turn, accelerate the aging and degenerative disease processes. Refrigeration of oils is vitally important. It would ideally be done in the stores but usually isn't. It is not standard practice in stores, homes or restaurants for oils to be refrigerated. Restaurants make matters worse with their frying, particularly deep fat frying. It is very damaging to the oil due to the extremely high temperatures used. Many foods served in restaurants are so prepared, and, *if* the restaurant is complying with health standards, the oil in the deep fat fryer may be changed only once a week.

I repeat the recommendation that only unrefined oils and oil products be used. This includes salad dressings, mayonnaise and peanut butter, all oil products that come in refined and unrefined form. Those commonly found in your supermarket are refined.

The body has a difficult time metabolizing fats if the liver is congested. And due to our eating habits and toxic exposure, most of us have congested livers. Many of us function on only 30% or less of liver capacity due to depletion of the sodium in the organ to neutralize acid toxins in the body. The liver is the largest organ in the body, and it performs a wide variety of functions, one of which is the manufacture of cholesterol. The healthy, unclogged liver will adjust its cholesterol production in accordance with the amount of fat consumed. Consumption of refined oils and hydrogenated ones are particularly damaging to the liver. Let's look more closely now at the hydrogenation process.

HYDROGENATION

Hydrogenated or "trans" fats are man-made. They do not spoil. Almost all processed foods today contain partially hydrogenated fats. Popular peanut butters that have a smooth, uniform texture and no oil floating on the top are an example. The jar of hydrogenated peanut butter you buy today will be just as "fresh" 60 years from now as it was when it was packaged — and just as dangerous to consume.

The hydrogenation process was not created by, nor for, the food industry. In 1912, a French scientist, Paul Sabatier, won the Nobel

Prize for succeeding in hydrogenating organic compounds. He wasn't looking for a way to prolong shelf life in food but rather for a way to make soap hard.

Sabatier succeeded in making the oil accept an extra bond of hydrogen by using nickel as a catalyst. This same process is used in the hydrogenation of oils in the food industry today. The fat, usually an unsaturated vegetable oil, is exposed to temperatures over 400 degrees, and small amounts of nickel are used to achieve the hydrogen bonding, changing it from a liquid to a solid form. Margarine is an example of a hydrogenated fat. It is generally thought to be unsaturated because it is made from vegetable oils that are unsaturated. However, once they have been through the hydrogenation process, they become super-saturated with hydrogen.

Once oil has gone through the process of hydrogenation, it is no longer an oil but a plastic, a celluloid. Oils are partially hydrogenated, for were they completely hydrogenated, they would form into hard plastic-like chips. In the words of John H.Tobe:

> Hydrogenated fat is nothing but sheer hard plastic, a new inorganic chemical compound that will not melt when you squeeze and rub it against your fingers, generating more than body heat. If these hydrogenated fats will not flow or at least break down at body temperature, then exactly what would you expect your bloodstream to do with these plastic particles?(5)

What your bloodstream does with these plastic particles is to retain them as obstructions to blood flow. They therefore become a significant factor in the development of coronary artery disease. It is no coincidence that heart disease increased with the introduction of hydrogenated fats in our diet. Homogenization is also a process that plays a significant role in heart disease and is discussed in chapter 11. Remember the time table: Americans were still fairly healthy in the first quarter of the 20th century. Rapid decline in health followed the introduction of food refining processes, one of the most harmful of which is hydrogenation.

Hydrogenated oil, like mineral oil, prevents the absorption of fat-soluble vitamins by binding with them in the body. Neither of these oils should be consumed, nor should mineral oil (baby oil) be rubbed on the skin, for it enters the bloodstream in that manner.

Hydrogenated oils are devoid of natural fat emulsifiers; they inhibit gallbladder function and promote inflammation. Hydrogenated products include most commercial peanut butter and baked goods, all margarine, shortening and processed cheeses. And once again, hydrogenated oil is an ingredient (though not necessarily appearing on the label) in most processed foods. These fats should be completely avoided. A *Lancet* medical study suggests that a high intake of trans fats may increase the risk of coronary death by 50-67%.[6] It is not known how much trans fat, if any, can be safely consumed, but many experts recommend limiting daily intake to two grams. Mary Enig, an expert on the subject of fats, believes that Americans are typically consuming a whopping 11-28 grams per day.[7] Due to recent findings indicating that trans-fatty acids raise serum levels of low density lipoproteins (LDL, the so-called "bad" cholesterol), the FDA is now developing new regulations mandating that trans-fatty acid content be listed on nutrition labels.

The body cannot process or utilize the trans fats created by the hydrogenation process. It is ironic that many people, even some doctors, still think eating margarine is healthier than eating butter because they believe the margarine to be unsaturated. The truth, of course, is that the margarine is much more saturated than butter. Butter, especially in its raw state, with the lipase enzyme intact, is to be far preferred over margarine. Raw butter can be purchased in many natural food stores, but note that it does have an expiration date, as it is made with raw, unpasteurized milk. Raw foods are generally to be preferred over cooked ones (and pasteurization is a form of cooking), for they are whole foods with their enzymes intact. The lipase enzyme, which breaks down fat, is not found in pasteurized milk, butter or cheese, but is present in these foods in their raw state. The American public consumes copious amounts of pasteurized dairy products. These products, lacking in the protease and lipase enzymes needed to break down proteins and fats respectively, are not properly digested, and their consumption results in putrefaction (and subsequent toxity), as well as elevated triglyceride and cholesterol levels in the body.

Hydrogenated fats are synthetic fats. Their production creates abnormal fatty acids.

ESSENTIAL FATTY ACIDS

When fats are eaten, they're broken down into glycerin and fatty acids (also known as vitamin F). Even if no fat is eaten, the body can make most of these fats from sugars. But two of them it cannot: **linoleic** and **linolenic acid.** These are the essential fatty acids (EFAs).

Animal studies show that EFA deficiencies result in eczema and sterility. Overweight, too, is linked with too little fat consumption, as Adelle Davis explained long ago:

> For three reasons, eating too little fat is probably a major cause of overweight. First, many seemingly fat persons are only waterlogged: An adequate diet, including salad dressing daily, often causes them to lose pounds. Second, it has been proved by what is known as the respiratory quotient that when the essential fatty acids are insufficiently supplied, the body changes sugar to fat much more rapidly than is normal; Dr. Bloor points out that it would seem as if the body were speedily trying to produce the missing nutrients.
>
> This quick change makes the blood sugar plunge downward, causing you to be as starved as a wolf; the chances are that you overeat and gain weight. Third, fats are more satisfying than any other foods. If you forego eating 100 calories of fat per meal, you usually become so hungry that you eat 500 calories of starch and/or sugar simply because you cannot resist them; unwanted pounds creep on...(8)

Earlier I mentioned the Omega-3 and Omega-6 fatty acids, forms of polyunsaturated fats. The EFA, linoleic acid, belongs to the Omega-6 family. From linoleic acid, gamma-linolenic acid (GLA) is derived. And from GLA, arachidonic acid is derived, though it can also be supplied exogenously through red meat. A second EFA, linolenic acid, gives rise to eicosapentaenoic acid (EPA) and docosahexaenoic acid (DHA), as depicted in chart 9A.

From DGLA, EPA, DHA and arachidonic acid are made the prostaglandins, which control so many vital functions of the body. EFA deficiencies can negatively impact prostaglandin production and therefore cause problems.

It is important to know that the processing of oils prevents the conversion of linoleic acid to GLA, and that Omega-3 EFAs are removed from refined foods to retard spoilage. Food processing therefore produces EFA deficiencies and imbalances. Due to our

Chart 9A

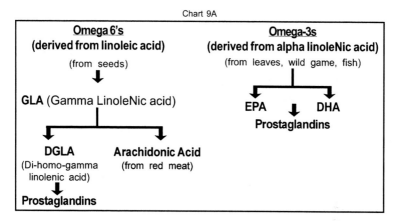

society's over-consumption of red meat, as well as an increase in the use of vegetable oils, the ratio of Omega-6 to Omega-3 fatty acids has increased tremendously. The problem and solution is well stated below by the editor of *Clinical Pearl News:*

> It is noted that the Western diet between the 1850s and 1995 has had a remarkable increase in Omega-6 to Omega-3 fatty acid ratio due to an increase in total fats and linoleic acid-rich vegetable oils. The Omega-6 to Omega-3 fatty acid ratio is believed to have risen from a 1:1 ratio to greater than a 10:1 ratio as fats from fish, wild game and leaves were replaced by increasing consumption of linoleic acid-rich oils from seeds. The increase in arachidonic acid and the reduction of EPA in the cell membranes leads to an over-production of inflammatory eicosanoids (a category of hormones which includes prostaglandins). These substances are related to chronic degenerative diseases that are so prevalent in Western culture. (Inflammatory conditions and depression may be lessened by reducing the arachidonic acid to EPA ratio). This can be done most simply by reduction of meat, eggs and dairy fat and the increase in consumption of fish, vegetables, flax seed and walnuts.(9)

The imbalance we've created becomes even more problematic when we consider that the body needs 50-100 times more EPA (an Omega-3 EFA) than GLA (an Omega-6).

It should be noted that the polyunsaturated fatty acids are extremely heat-sensitive. They spoil very readily. These oils should therefore never be used for cooking. Cook instead with unrefined olive oil or coconut oil. These are both quality oils that have a high resistance to heat. Although coconut oil received a lot of bad press at one time (from the vegetable oil industry), the fact of the matter is that it has many healthful qualities. All of the tropical oils (palm, palm kernel and coconut) contain large quantities of lauric acid. Lauric acid is a fatty acid which has strong anti-fungal and anti-microbial properties. These are very stable oils that don't require refrigeration. They can be kept at room temperature for many months without going rancid.

CARBOHYDRATES

All the plants we eat, whether fruits, vegetables or grains, are carbohydrates. Sugars and starches are included in this category. The body converts all sugars and starches to glucose (blood sugar). You will recall that ATP (the fuel for the electrical generator, the sodium/potassium pump) is made up primarily of glucose and oxygen. Of all the nutrients, carbohydrates are the best source of glucose. They are the chief source of energy for all body functions and muscular exertion, providing us with immediately available calories for energy by producing heat in the body when carbon in the system unites with oxygen in the bloodstream.

Carbohydrates can be manufactured in the body from some amino acids and the glycerol component of fats. Therefore, there is no established RDA. Carbohydrates are necessary to assist in the digestion and assimilation of other foods. Those found in fruits and vegetables help reduce the need for protein.

As previously stated, refined grains have had their fiber and germ and many of their vitamins and minerals removed. Some, but not all of the B vitamins removed during milling, are replaced in the "enriching" process. B vitamin deficiencies are therefore created as a result of the widespread consumption of refined carbohydrates. If the B vitamins are absent, carbohydrate combustion cannot take place, and indigestion and symptoms of nausea and heartburn occur. Americans take in large quantities of refined carbohydrates and cannot properly digest them, not only because of B vitamin deficiencies but also due to improperly combined foods. A cardinal rule of food combining is to avoid eating starchy carbohydrates and proteins at the same meal. Combinations like cheese and bread, milk and cereal, potatoes and meat, and eggs and toast are as American as apple pie — and just as difficult to digest! Proteins require an acid digestive secretion, while carbohydrates call for an alkaline one. We all know what happens when acid meets alkaline — The fluids become neutralized, and nothing gets properly digested. The protein putrefies. The carbohydrate ferments. This means they rot in the body, creating toxins that are acid in nature.

We would do well to replace refined carbohydrates with complex carbohydrates (starches). These take longer to digest than simple sugars (fruits, sucrose and other concentrated sweeteners such as honey, molasses, maple syrup). It is important to realize, however, that some complex carbs have a higher glycemic index than do simple sugars. This means they are more quickly converted to blood sugar in the bloodstream, giving rise to a rapid increase in insulin release. The glycemic index rating for rice cakes is 133 (pure glucose is 100) and for whole wheat it's 100, while peaches and apples have ratings of only 29 and 39, respectively, even though they are simple sugars. Consuming high glycemic index foods (such as carrots) by themselves triggers an immediate insulin response, which is soon followed by a rapid drop in blood sugar. Choosing foods with a low glycemic rating will help us achieve sustained energy — and appetite control. Refer to the abbreviated glycemic index (Chart 9B).

Consuming any carbohydrate, simple or complex, with a high or low glycemic index rating will result in secretion of insulin from the pancreas. This hormone drives sugar into the cells, lowering blood sugar levels. What's left is stored in the liver and muscles as glycogen. Once these rather limited storehouses are full, the remainder is stored as body fat. Insulin therefore does two things: It lowers blood sugar and stores glucose as fat.

Just as insulin is secreted when we consume carbohydrates, another hormone, glucagon, is released when we eat protein. Insulin and glucose are inversely paired hormones, which means when one is high, the other is low. While insulin lowers blood sugar, glucagon raises it. While insulin stores fat, glucagon mobilizes fat from storage depots so it can be burned as fuel. Consuming too many carbs in relationship to protein (a high carbohydrate/protein ratio) will result in a continual insulin response, leading to low blood sugar initially (diabetes ultimately) and weight gain.

Clearly, to restore hormonal balance, we need to lower the carbohydrate/protein ratio. As already mentioned, this is best done by decreasing the carbs rather than increasing the already excessive protein in the SAD. By cutting down on the intake of carbs, insulin/

Abbreviated Glycemic Index

High Glycemic Index (70% - 100%+)

Puffed rice and wheat
Corn flakes
Maltose
Millet
Instant white rice
Tofu ice cream substitute
Glucose
White bread
Whole wheat bread
Carrots
Parsnips
Barley (whole meal)
Apricots
Corn chips
Rolled oats
Honey
Rice (white and brown)
Bananas
Corn
White potato
Ripe mango
Ripe papaya
Kidney beans
Buckwheat

Low Glycemic Index (10-40%)

Apples
Black-eyed peas
Chick peas
Pears
Ice cream
Milk
Lentils
Fructose
Plums
Peaches
Grapefruit
Cherries
Soybeans
Peanuts

Note: the glycemic index of an individual food can be lowered by consuming it with other foods, especially fatty foods.

Moderate Glycemic Index (40-70%)

Raisins
Bulgur wheat
Spaghetti (white and whole wheat)
Pinto beans
Macaroni
Beets
Rye
Couscous
Apple juice/apple sauce
Sucrose
Potato chips
Barley (coarse)
Lactose
Yam
Sweet potato
Beans (lima, butter, navy)
Peas
Oranges and Orange juice

(Chart 9B)

glucagon levels can be balanced. Barry Sears maintains that a diet whose caloric composition consists of 40% carbs, 30% protein and 30% fat will provide the desired hormonal balance. To maintain this balance, the 40/30/30 intake must be kept up at every meal and at snack time. This, he maintains, is the key to being "in the zone" and thereby regulating eicosanoid production and normalizing virtually all physiological processes. Balanced macronutrient consumption is especially beneficial to cardiac function and for the regulation of weight and blood sugar levels.

In order for the whole system to be at its best, there must also be a balance between glucose and oxygen. When this balance is off, the body goes into a state of stress, with a resulting strain on the endocrine system, leading to glandular exhaustion. All sugars provide glucose to the body. However, some are more usable than others, more assimilable. All man-made sugars — those extracted and concentrated from food sources and those made from chemicals — are difficult for the body to utilize. While they provide abundant glucose, they are lacking in the nutrients needed to utilize the glucose. What follows is a comprehensive listing of sugars and other sweeteners. This information comes from Earl Mindell's *Unsafe at Any Meal:*

SUCROSE - table sugar. A disaccharide (double sugar – glucose + fructose). It has no nutrients, requires B vitamins to assimilate, comes from cane or beet sugar.

GLUCOSE - the body's blood sugar. A monosaccharide, found in most fruits. It is readily assimilated by the body.

DEXTROSE - made from corn starch. It is a monosaccharide that is chemically identical to glucose.

FRUCTOSE (levulose) - found in fruits, but many fruits are mainly sucrose. It is absorbed more slowly than sucrose, is highly refined and devoid of nutrients, even when derived from natural sources.

MALTOSE - a non-nutritious disaccharide made from the malting of grains.

LACTOSE - glucose + galactose. It is as non-nutritive as all other refined sugars but feeds the beneficial intestinal bacteria.

BROWN SUGAR - white, refined sugar with molasses coloring.

RAW or TURBINADO SUGAR - is packaged at 96% sucrose (table sugar is 99%) and has no nutritive benefit.

BLACKSTRAP MOLASSES - the liquid that remains after beet and cane sugar have been thoroughly processed and the sucrose has been removed. It is still 65% sucrose and contains minor but useful amounts of iron, calcium, potassium and B vitamins. The darker the molasses, the more nutritious.

HONEY – has the highest sugar content of all sweeteners (64 calories per teaspoon as compared to refined sugar's 48). It has small amounts of potassium, calcium and phosphorous and contains natural enzymes and pollen if unheated. Some varieties have been found to contain carcinogens that the bees have extracted from flowers sprayed with cancer-causing chemicals. Some bees are fed sugar.

MAPLE SYRUP – 65% sucrose. In commercial preparation, sap may be gathered in lead-soldered buckets and formaldehyde pellets used to keep the tap holes from healing and to increase the sap flow. Chemical anti-foaming agents are sometimes used.

MALT SYRUPS – made from several grains, they contain mainly maltose and glucose. They are nutritionally superior but not as sweet as maple syrups. Some have added sweetness from commercial corn syrup, which is industrially refined glucose. Barley malt syrup is the least sweet but the most wholesome. These syrups are usually not made from organic grains.

XYLITOL – although found naturally in berries, fruits and mush-rooms, it is generally extracted from birch cellulose. It is considered a carbohydrate alcohol and has some value as sugar but is metabolized differently. Large doses in long-term feeding studies have caused liver, kidney and brain disturbances in humans.

SORBITOL – half as sweet as sucrose. It occurs naturally in fruits, berries, algae and seaweeds. It is made industrially from hydrogen and commercial glucose (corn syrup). It is absorbed slowly, and large doses have a laxative effect.

MANNITOL – occurs naturally in beets, celery, olives, but is made commercially in the same way as sorbitol. It is half as sweet as sugar and produces diarrhea at lower levels than does sorbitol.

ASPARTAME (Nutrasweet and Equal) – composed of two amino acids, phenylalinine and aspartic acid, it is 200 times sweeter than sugar. Its use has been implicated in numerous disorders ranging from nausea and headaches to seizures, rashes, blindness and brain damage. (More information in the next section)

SACCHARIN – a non-caloric petroleum derivative, it is 300-500 times sweeter than sugar. It is not absorbed by the body, but has been linked with bladder cancer in laboratory animals.

CYCLAMATE – a non-caloric sweetener, 30 times sweeter than sugar, it has been implicated in causing testicular atrophy and chromosome damage. It has been banned in the U.S. and in Britain.

These last three, aspartame, saccharin and cyclamate are totally man-made.

As you can see from this discussion, there are drawbacks to all of the sweeteners listed by Mindell. Our best source of glucose is organically grown whole foods. Mineral-rich fruits and vegetables are very sweet-tasting. Those grown on impoverished soils have a bitter taste. Grain sprouted to 1" in length is as sweet as candy. We would do well to eliminate or significantly decrease our use of exogenous sweeteners, both natural and artificial. They are too rich for the body.

ASPARTAME

Aspartame is one of the most widely used — and insidious – – of the artificial sweeteners. It enjoys the official endorsement of some very prestigious groups, including the American Dietetics Association, the American Medical Association and the American Diabetes

Association. Their endorsement has more to do with politics and economics, however, than with health, for aspartame is a drug, not a food additive. It was discovered by a scientist from G.D. Searle, a drug company. FDA approval of the drug in 1974 was based solely upon tests provided by Searle. That approval was later rescinded because of safety issues, then reinstated despite objections from respected scientists. Searle and Nutrasweet are now owned by Monsanto Co. (the rBGH people — see chapter 11).

Worldwide aspartame sales exceed $1 billion yearly, 700 million of which is U.S. revenue. Five thousand products now contain the chemical — diet sodas, Kool-aid, jello, teas, cocoa, juices, frozen desserts, puddings, cakes, cereals, candies, etc., and the patent has now expired, opening the way for wider use. It's even found in vitamins and medicines. In 1985, 800 million pounds of aspartame soft drinks were consumed in this country. Aspartame is now available in more than 90 countries worldwide. In addition to the amino acids phenylalanine and aspartic acid, it contains methanol (methyl alcohol), a deadly metabolic poison that is converted in the body to formaldehyde and formic acid (known to cause cancer, genetic mutations and birth defects) before being ultimately broken down into carbon dioxide. Methyl alcohol is eliminated by the body five times more slowly than is ethyl alcohol found in alcoholic beverages. Because of this, it is cumulative in the system. Methanol is listed as a "human poison by ingestion" in *Sax's Dangerous Properties of Industrial Materials.* It is toxic to the nervous system, especially the optic nerve, so its ingestion can lead to progressive loss of sight. There are numerous other symptoms of methanol poisoning that do not show up immediately.

Aspartame breaks down into methanol within one hour of ingestion. Heat speeds up the process. Nonetheless, aspartame was approved for use in baked goods, cocoa, tea and other heated products in 1993.

Phenylalanine, in large doses, is toxic to the brain. It can cause mental retardation and seizures in people with phenylketonuria (PKU), a genetic disorder. An estimated 4.5 million people have one of the two genes necessary for PKU. While they won't develop the disease, they may be sensitive to phenylalanine and not know it. Aspartic acid by itself, according to literature from the Aspartame Consumer Safety Network, is a neurotoxin, as well as a known cause of endocrine disorders and brain tumors. It destroys brain cells and is especially hazardous to the developing central nervous system of young children.

Aspartame has the distinction of having more consumer complaints registered against it than any other product in history (7,000). Reported adverse effects include:

abdominal pain	dry eyes (lack of tears)
aggression	anxiety
bloating	blood pressure instability
chronic fatigue	death
depression	diarrhea
drowsiness	edema (fluid retention)
eye pain	hearing impairment
irritability	heart palpitations
itching	increase in infection
nausea	numbness
phobias	ringing in the ears
sleepiness	shortness of breath
slurring of speech	tingling
unsteadiness	urinary tract burning
urinary frequency	migraine headaches
perceptual disorders	memory loss
weight gain	mania
seizures	

The above are just some of the 92 documented symptoms caused by aspartame use.

Dr. William Campbell Douglass, M.D., reports in the 3/96 edition of his newsletter *Second Opinion* that the National Institute of Health has published a report listing 167 reasons why aspartame should not be used. He also informs us that aspartame was "once listed by the Pentagon as a possible biochemical warfare weapon..."

Flying Safety, the official Air Force safety magazine, and *Navy Physiology,* the Navy's flight magazine, have both published warnings about using aspartame while flying, as a significant number of pilots have experienced aspartame-induced seizures and perceptual disorders. Mary Nash Stoddard, who founded the Aspartame Consumer Safety Network, formed a Pilots Hotline, which had received over 500 pilot-related calls as of 11/95.

For more information regarding the problems associated with aspartame, contact the Aspartame Safety Network, P.O. Box 780634,

Dallas, TX   75378, (214)352-4268. They put out an excellent video, "Aspartame — the Deadly Deception."

FRUCTOSE

Many health-oriented individuals see fructose as a healthy alternative to aspartame and sucrose. Because of its low glycemic index rating, it has often been recommended for diabetics. However, animal studies indicate that it seriously interferes with copper metabolism — to the extent that collagen and elastin can't form in growing animals. The result is hypertrophy of the heart and liver in young animals and resorption of litters in adult females.

There's a great deal of fructose, in the form of high fructose corn syrup, consumed today — three times as much as was consumed in 1980. The sweetener is frequently found in "health" foods.

Because the liver is the only organ in the body that can metabolize fructose, a high consumption of it seriously stresses this vital organ. Due to the liver's role in sugar metabolism, fructose should be avoided by diabetics.[10]

STEVIA

An ideal sweetener is a South American herb stevia. It is 30 to 40 times sweeter than sugar and has no known harmful effects. On the contrary: It has been found to actually help stabilize blood sugar levels and does not cause tooth decay. It is now available in powdered and liquid form in health food stores.

Although very sweet, stevia is virtually non-caloric. Ironically, however, the FDA does not permit it to be marketed as a "sweetener." In fact, in 1991, they banned the import of the herb into the U.S. That year armed federal marshals actually seized one Texas distributor's shipment from Brazil.

Why did the FDA make this ideal sweetener illegal? It would appear that the makers of more expensive chemical sweeteners didn't want competition from an herb that cannot be patented. The FDA denied GRAS status (Generally Recognized As Safe) to stevia, and by so doing, placed it in the "food additive" category. This placement requires that a product undergo extensive scientific study before being marketed.

Despite the FDA's constraints on stevia, the way was cleared for it to enter the U.S. market in 1994 with passage of the Dietary Supplement Health and Education Act (DSHEA). This legislation allowed stevia to become a recognized "dietary supplement" by the fall of 1995. Its use as a sweetener is still prohibited, however. For this reason, it cannot be added as such to commercial foods or beverages. It *is* available in health food stores in whole leaf powder, extract and liquid form, however. *The Stevia Cookbook* by Gates and Sahelian (Avery Publishing, 1999) provides over 100 recipes using this sweet substance that may not be called a sweetener.

SUCROSE

Table sugar is sucrose. Sucrose is cane or beet sugar. As Dr. Mindell notes, it contains no nutrients (except calories) and requires B vitamins for assimilation. So, sugar consumption makes extra demands on the body's already depleted supply of B vitamins.

In 1870, Americans consumed 11 teaspoons of sugar daily. A hundred years later, in 1970, we were taking in 32 teaspoons, almost a threefold increase. In 1980, the rate of sugar consumption was up to 38 teaspoons per person per day. By 1995, sugar consumption in this country was up to 170# per person per year (compared to 10# in 1821). This amounts to ¼ the total average caloric intake.(11) From where are we getting all of this sugar? Much of it is hidden in our food. Start reading labels. Know that anything ending in "ose" is some form of sugar. Beware of products labeled "unsweetened," as they may have sugar added to restore them to a "normal" level of sweetness. More than 50% of the sugar we now consume comes from high fructose corn syrup (making corn a common allergen). A good portion also comes from artificial sweeteners.

There are many harmful effects of sugar consumption. In her book, *Lick the Sugar Habit,* Nancy Appleton, Ph.D., discusses the relationship between sugar consumption and the development of allergies. Because certain minerals (chromium, manganese, magnesium, copper, cobalt and zinc) are needed to metabolize sugar, and these minerals are largely discarded in the refining process, the body is forced to rob its own storehouses, depleting mineral reserves and interfering with mineral balance when sugar is consumed. This depletion and imbalance also interferes with enzyme function (since minerals are the catalysts for many enzyme activities) so that foods are not properly digested. When undigested food particles enter the bloodstream, the body views them as foreign invaders and launches an immune response, giving rise to an allergic reaction. For this reason, the foods to which most people are allergic (milk, corn, wheat, chocolate, etc.) are those that are typically eaten with sugar. Because protein digestion is problematic anyway — and is so extremely important — proteins should never be consumed with sugar. Appleton summarizes the problem succinctly:

> Through the combined effects of mineral imbalance, allergic re-action and phagocytic suppression, sugar can destroy the immune system and slowly but surely lead to degenerative disease.(12)

Sugar deranges the apestat mechanism so that the body's inherent wisdom regarding food selection becomes impaired. We then build addictive patterns, craving more sugar rather than needed nutrients. Sugar displaces other foods in the sense that it occupies space that could otherwise be filled with nutritious foods. As already mentioned, it robs the body of B vitamins needed to metabolize it. Excess sugar intake also leads to increased urinary excretion of calcium, contributing to deficiency of this mineral. Since sugar is acid-forming, intake of large amounts contributes to the creation of acidosis in the system. Demineralization of muscles, organs and bones (to buffer the acid) follows if an abundance of alkaline minerals is not supplied in the diet. Sugar also destroys vitamin C and has been linked with a build-up of cholesterol in the blood.

It has been found that people with moderately severe atherosclerosis usually have mild hypoglycemia, and those with moderate and severe diabetes have especially severe atherosclerois. In other words, the worse the blood sugar disorder, the higher the cholesterol level. It has been demonstrated that many diabetics have more than ample amounts of insulin in their blood. According to the late Nathan Pritikin, it is the presence of excessive levels of fat that prevents the insulin from getting into the cell system. Since life begins and ends at the cellular level, unless we can get nutrients into the cells where they belong, they will not nourish the body. Blood sugar disorders themselves are, in part, a consequence of over-consumption of sugar.

BLOOD SUGAR DISORDERS

The brain uses 50% of all available glucose in the blood. Changes in blood sugar level affect the brain and therefore affect behavior. Most of us know that diabetes is a condition of too much sugar in the blood (hyperglycemia) and not enough insulin (hypoinsulinism). Insulin is the hormone that makes it possible for glucose to enter the cells and be converted into energy. Each time we consume sugar, the pancreas is called upon to secrete insulin. That insulin will drive about 30% of the sugar consumed into the cells. The other 70% is stored in the liver as glycogen.

Insulin supplementation (oral or injectable) is the medical treatment of choice for diabetes. The exogenous insulin forces the cell to accept glucose, and sugar levels are thereby controlled. Insulin supplementation is by no means a cure for diabetes, however.

To better understand diabetes, we need to look at the mechanism of action of its precursor, hypoglycemia (low blood sugar). At first glance, it would seem that diabetes and low blood sugar are opposites, for one involves too much sugar in the blood, the other too little. In reality, however, hypoglycemia precedes diabetes. It was first identified in 1924, when Dr. Seal Harris noticed non-diabetics who were showing signs of insulin shock: nervousness, tiredness, cold sweats, convulsions, fainting. The standard test for measuring blood sugar levels at that time called for blood to be analyzed at hourly intervals for three consecutive hours after a fasting patient was given glucose orally. By extending this test up to six hours, Dr. Harris found that patients who may have shown normal (80-120) readings initially would often experience a drop in the blood sugar level in the final hours of the test. When the blood sugar level fell below 80, the condition was termed "hypoglycemia." It was further found through this extended glucose tolerance test that some patients who showed blood sugar levels above normal initially (in the diabetic range) would dip into the hypoglycemic range in the final hours of the test. This condition was termed "dysinsulinism." It is best treated in the same manner as hypoglycemia. Since the condition cannot be detected with the standard test, and such a test is likely to yield false results, its use could lead to a patient being misdiagnosed as diabetic. Administration of insulin to such a patient would certainly create problems, for when he is in his hypoglycemic phase, his body is already producing too much insulin. To clarify, let's look at the terms:

HYPOglycemia = HYPERinsulinism = Low Blood Sugar
HYPERglycemia = HYPOinsulinism = High Blood Sugar (Diabetes)

To better understand the causal relationship between these apparently opposite conditions, let us consider what happens when we eat. When we take in sugar (and/or caffeine and alcohol), the pancreas secretes insulin. When we consume these items frequently in large quantities, we are making rather tall demands upon the pancreas. It is therefore kept quite busy secreting insulin and, after a time, goes into hyperactivity. When the pancreas secretes too much insulin, we have a condition of too little sugar in the blood. Now, remember the sugar that was originally stored in the liver as glycogen? When the blood sugar level begins to drop during periods when we are not eating, it is the job of the liver to convert some of this glycogen back into sugar to be supplied to the blood to raise the blood sugar level. However, as has been previously discussed, most of us have impaired liver function. When the blood sugar level starts to drop, the hypothalamus, whose job it is to monitor internal body functions, directs the adrenal glands to secrete adrenaline or epinepherine which triggers the liver to convert its glycogen to sugar. This is what is supposed to happen. A breakdown in communications between these organs, as well as a liver impairment, can result in hypoglycemia going unchecked, however. So, low blood sugar has a lot to do with the liver, not just the pancreas.

Most people today, certainly those on the SAD, are hypoglycemic but just don't know it. And hypoglycemia is the first step toward diabetes. Remember: An organ goes first into hyperfunction and then into hypofunction. Over a period of time, the overworked pancreas may, indeed, decrease its insulin production, at which time we have adult onset diabetes. Diabetes is the result of a severely dysfunctional pancreas. But remember, too, what Pritikin pointed out: Many diabetics have sufficient insulin in their blood; it is simply not getting to the cellular level due to obstruction by fatty deposits. Pritikin gave examples of diabetics whose condition improved significantly after eliminating fat from their diets. The link between high cholesterol and blood sugar disorders is well established.

Sub-clinical hypoglycemia can produce such symptoms as irritability, anxiety, unstable temper, moodiness, headache and fatigue — a familiar set of symptoms, often misdiagnosed. Hypoglycemia is an underlying condition in asthma, allergies, hay fever, rheumatic fever, ulcers and in most cases of mental illness.

The standard medical treatment for hypoglycemia is dietary control, with recommendation of frequent ingestion of high protein foods. This may make us feel better due to the stimulation provided by the protein, but it is not the best long-term solution. As has already been discussed, a high protein diet causes putrefaction in the colon and production of poisonous by-products that cause trapped plasma protein. For the hypoglycemic, the 40/30/30 diet or the *ProVita Plan* is, I believe, a better choice.

Chromium is needed to metabolize blood sugar. It works with insulin, facilitating the entry of glucose into the cells. Without chromium, the tissues become insensitive to insulin. The lower the total body chromium level, the worse the glucose metabolism. White sugar in the diet contributes to the loss of chromium from the body and consequent deficiency. Pure chromium is poorly absorbed by the body, which produces its own in a special molecular structure called GTF (Glucose Tolerance Factor) made up of cysteine, glycine, glutamic acid, niacin and chromium. Yeast is an excellent source of GTF, but is contraindicated for patients with Candida albicans. Brewer's yeast is popular in health circles. However, it is a high stress protein if consumed in any but small amounts, according to Stuart Wheelwright.

Dr. William Philpot in *Brain Allergies* has observed that food allergies, gone long undetected, can produce behavioral abnormalities, even psychoses. He discusses methods of identifying food allergens and has found that any food, regardless of glucose content, to which a person is allergic, can cause a disturbance in blood sugar level. Food and environmental allergies have become widespread. The allergic reaction is an autoimmune response that, ironically, can be attributed, at least in part, to the use of allopathic medicines, particularly antibiotics. Dr. Reckeweg *(Homotoxicology)* you'll recall, tells us that molecules of the drug, along with molecules of the bacterial endotoxins (from the remains of dead microorganisms), become encoded in the body's own protein, and the immune response is therefore launched against self, as well as nonself.

In summary then, as regards macronutrients, the substitution of unrefined complex carbohydrates and those with a low glycemic index for simple sugars and carbs with a high glycemic index, the avoidance of hydrogenated fats and high stress proteins, as well as the gradual introduction of raw foods into the diet, is recommended. Where fats are concerned, small amounts of unrefined oils are essential to the body. In their extracted form, these oils oxidize (turn rancid) rapidly and therefore should be used with discretion. Extracted oils — both of the saturated and unsaturated variety — can be a burden to the body, especially if they are refined and therefore lacking in the enzymes needed to digest them. With oils, as with all other food products, it is most desirable that they be consumed as an integral part of the whole food.

The diet can more closely approximate the ideal as alkaline reserves and vitality are restored to the body. Whether we are dealing with hypoglycemia, diabetes, heart disease, cancer or arthritis, the road to reversal of the degenerative disease process is the same. Violation of nature's laws can result in a myriad of conditions, while restoration of health is achieved by obedience to those laws, which remain constant — regardless of the variety of symptoms expressed.

CHAPTER 10

More Essential Nutrients
(Vitamins, Minerals, Water)

*"If you take a vitamin pill in the morning,
your body spends the afternoon looking for
the rest of the carrot."*
                              Annemarie Colbin

The last of the six essential nutrients are vitamins, minerals and water. All are natural components of food. All are essential to our survival. There are many issues tied in with each of these topics. This chapter will focus on some of the major ones.

VITAMINS

The *Concise American Heritage Dictionary* defines a vitamin as follows:

> Any of relatively complex organic substances occurring naturally in plant and animal tissue and essential in small amounts for metabolic processes.

The *Merriam-Webster Dictionary* gives the following definition:

> Any of the various organic substances that are essential in tiny amounts to most animals and some plants and are mostly obtained from foods.

Please note the last four words, "mostly obtained from foods." The classic description of a vitamin is a substance that is essential to life and can be obtained *only* from outside sources, from food. According to this definition then, a substance may not be regarded as a vitamin if it can be synthesized within the body from the elements obtained from food sources. It has been found, however, that certain substances, already classified as vitamins, can be synthesized in the body under optimal conditions. B vitamins are an example. Given the proper balance of beneficial bacteria in the intestines, many of these can be produced internally. Therefore, our concept of a vitamin is changing.

Note that each of the dictionary definitions states that vitamins are found in living things and are essential to their existence in *small* or *tiny* amounts. What is spoken of here is the vitamin in its *natural* form, as it was created by nature, as an integral part of food. The only vitamins that may truly be considered natural are those that remain attached to their food source. Here they exist with other elements with which they work in harmony, synergistically. In the form of food, nature has provided us with a correct balance of elements, provided the soil from which the food has come is not depleted of nutrients. Soil depletion is a clear and present reality that has given impetus to the trend toward organic gardening. Organic produce is far more nutrient-rich than its non-organic, commercially grown counterpart. (See chart 10A).

We refer to A, C, D and E as vitamins, but to B as a complex, giving the impression that it is the only one of the vitamins containing more than one element. This is not accurate. Years ago, Dr. Royal Lee taught us the difference between a natural complex and a synthetic, *crystalline* vitamin. All vitamins, as they occur naturally, are part of a complex. "These vitamin complexes consist of enzymes, coenzymes, antioxidant and trace mineral activators."(1) The isolated vitamin portion of a complex is what is referred to as a crystalline vitamin. When this portion of the complex is separated from its naturally-occurring companion elements, its biological activity is virtually destroyed, for it must recombine with the other members of the complex before it can assume its nutrient function. As an example, what we refer to as vitamin C, ascorbic acid, is the crystalline element in the vitamin C complex, just one of many elements of the complex (see chart 10-B). Ascorbic acid can't be utilized by the body unless the other elements of the C complex are present in the body and these elements successfully hook up with the crystalline portion before it's lost in the urine.

When the trace mineral activator of a vitamin complex is not present in the body, the crystalline vitamin cannot be utilized. The mineral activator in the C complex is tyrosinase (organic copper). Ascorbic acid cannot be utilized by the body of one who is deficient in this element. Selenium activates the E complex, and manganese activates the B complex.

High potency crystalline vitamins can actually be harmful to the body in that they can induce deficiencies of the co-factors leached to utilize the crystalline portion of the complex. A co-factor of the vitamin C complex that became very popular recently is pycnogenol. Pycnogenol is one of over **4000** flavonoids (plant pigments) that serves an antioxidant function, protecting against free radical damage. Continual use of large doses of this flavonoid can deplete the body of other C complex co-factors. When they are expended, the pycnogenol itself will not be well utilized.

In 1939, Albert von Szent-Gyorgi, who won the Nobel Prize for discovering that vitamin C cured scurvy, wrote about a colleague of his who cured an infection through use of a paprika preparation

CHART 10A
VARIATIONS IN MINERAL CONTENT IN VEGETABLES
Firman E. Bear Report, Rutgers University*

	PERCENTAGE OF DRY WEIGHT		MILLEQUIVALENTS PER 100 GRAMS DRY WEIGHT				TRACE ELEMENTS PARTS PER MILLION DRY MATTER				
	Total Ash or Mineral Matter	Phosphorus	Calcium	Magnesium	Potassium	Sodium	Boron	Manganese	Iron	Copper	Cobalt
SNAP BEANS											
ORGANIC	10.45	0.36	40.5	60.0	99.7	8.6	73	60	227	69.0	0.26
INORGANIC	4.04	0.22	15.5	14.8	29.1	0.0	10	2	10	3.0	0.00
CABBAGE											
ORGANIC	10.38	0.38	60.0	43.6	148.3	20.4	42	13	94	48.0	0.15
INORGANIC	6.12	0.18	17.5	13.6	33.7	0.8	7	2	20	0.4	0.00
LETTUCE											
ORGANIC	24.48	0.43	71.0	49.3	176.5	12.2	37	169	516	60.0	0.19
INORGANIC	7.01	0.22	16.0	13.1	53.0	0.0	6	1	9	3.0	0.00
TOMATOES											
ORGANIC	14.2	0.35	23.0	59.2	148.3	6.5	36	68	1938	53.0	0.63
INORGANIC	6.07	0.16	4.5	4.5	58.8	0.0	3	1	1	0.0	0.00
SPINACH											
ORGANIC	28.56	0.52	96.0	203.9	237.0	69.5	88	117	1584	32.0	0.25
INORGANIC	12.38	0.27	47.5	46.9	84.6	0.8	12	1	19	0.3	0.20

*This report is not recent. It is over 50 years old.

CHART 10B

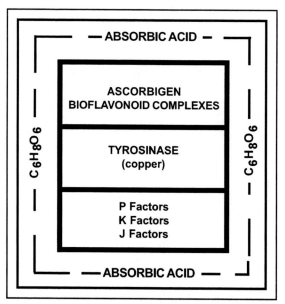

Vitamin C Complex

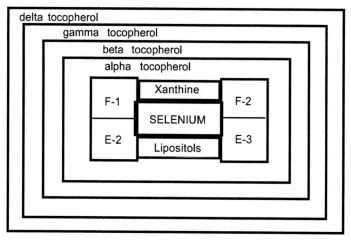

Vitamin E Complex

Above are what Dr. Richard Murray describes as the "functional architecture" of the vitamin C and vitamin E complexes in his "Applications in Human Nutrition" manual.

that contained much ascorbic acid. When he tried to produce the same effect with a similar condition, however, using pure ascorbic acid, he failed. Why? Because the ascorbic acid lacked the vital co-factors necessary to activate the ascorbic acid and allow healing to occur. "[Natural] vitamins are living enzyme complexes that naturally produce biochemical reactions in the human body, [while] synthetic vitamins are chemicals that produce pharmacological (drug) reactions in the body."(2) Because synthetic vitamins have drug-like effects, they can be dangerous when taken in large doses. I'll explore this fact more thoroughly, giving a surprising example, in the next chapter.

We hear a lot today about phytochemicals — plant chemicals. These phytochemicals contain the co-factors needed to activate crystalline vitamins. It may be said that phytochemicals and vitamins (the crystalline portion of the complex) activate each other. For this reason, vitamin complexes, as they occur in whole foods, have a healing power that is superior to that of synthetic vitamin fractions, regardless of their potency.(3)

Some recent studies have shown that certain antioxidants, like vitamins C and E and beta carotene, have failed to produce the therapeutic effect once claimed for them in fighting cancer. Why? Because these studies were done using only the antioxidant portion of the vitamin complex. The other vital co-factors were missing, reducing the therapeutic effect.

Antioxidants protect the plant in which they're found by preventing oxidation and other forms of destruction. Tocopherol is the antioxidant portion of the vitamin E complex. Other portions of the complex include xanthine, phospholipids, sex hormone precursors and lipositols(4), better known today as "tocotrienols." Tocopherol is not vitamin E, just as ascorbic acid is not vitamin C. They are but portions of their respective complexes. The potency of these vitamins, in the absence of their co-factors, is diminished regardless of how many milligrams or units of the vitamin they contain. Natural forms of the vitamin E complex lose up to 99% of their potency when separated from their natural co-factors, which serve as synergists. In fact, it has been established that purified vitamin E (tocopherols) in high unit doses actually reverses its effect and produces the same symptoms as a deficiency. This information comes from Dr. Bruce West, who also tells us that "synthetic vitamins are chemicals of one isolated portion of a vitamin fraction, and that fraction is not the same as found in nature. It is rather a mirror image that is identical but reversed."(5)

A vitamin complex contains enzymes, co-enzyme activators, antioxidant protective factors, amino acids, trace elements and other synergistic factors, *no doubt some not yet discovered.* For this reason, synthetic vitamins do not and cannot have the same effect as naturally-occurring ones.

Of the less than twenty vitamins discovered so far and believed to be active in human nutrition, most have been isolated and made available in tablet or capsule form in mega potencies. Many are labeled "all natural." If, as our definitions indicate, vitamins occur naturally in nature in only small or tiny amounts, how, you might wonder, can a high potency vitamin, such as a 500 mg. tablet of vitamin C be "all natural?" The answer is that it cannot be all natural in the sense that it came strictly from a food source, or else it would be larger than a golf ball! Your 500 mg. tablet of vitamin C may have the natural vitamin (from food sources) *in* it, but it is most assuredly composed primarily of ascorbic acid, the synthetic form of the vitamin. How then can such a product legally be labeled "all natural?" Easy: Who says "all natural" means the vitamin comes exclusively from food sources? Many who label their products "all natural" are operating within the context of a much broader definition of the word "natural." All life on this planet which science recognizes as organic is based on the property of carbon. Carbon occurs in many inorganic compounds as well. It is the primary element upon which life as we know it is based. In this corner of the universe, we live in carbon bodies. That which is "natural" to us is that which is carbon-based. In a very broad sense then, synthetic vitamins can be considered "all natural" since they have a coal tar base. Unbelievable as it may seem, the FDA allows anything containing only 5% natural ingredients to be called 100% natural!

In the natural vs. synthetic controversy, the pro-synthetic argument is made that both forms of the vitamin are chemically identical. The pro-natural side says yes, *but* the vitamin, in its natural form, is found in a whole food that contains other elements that are essential to the proper activity of the vitamin. Extracting the single vitamin and greatly increasing its potency through the addition of its synthetic counterpart disrupts nature's balance of elements, tipping the scales in favor of the crystalline vitamin portion, with little or none of the synergistic co-factors being provided. We may well be correcting one deficiency while simultaneously creating others. Science is forever looking for the "active ingredient" in the products of nature. Could it be that the curative power of whole food lies instead in its very wholeness? It would appear to be so. Recall the words "small" and "tiny" used in the definitions quoted at the beginning of this chapter. We live in a society that promotes the idea that "more is better," which is not necessarily so, as the system of homeopathic medicine proves. Whole foods have both a *synergistic* and a *molecular* structure. When single nutrients such as vitamins are extracted from food, the synergistic structure is destroyed. The isolated vitamin becomes a single chemical, lacking in life force and difficult for the body to utilize. Although natural and synthetic vitamins are chemically identical, it has been established that the atoms in a synthetic product rotate differently than the atoms of a natural one, and the natural product has a more dynamic energy pattern.

Where there is a demonstrated deficiency of a specific vitamin, it may be useful to supply it in a concentrated form until the natural balance of elements can be restored through diet. However, synthetic supplements can add to the toxic burden of the body. Even truly natural supplements can be a dross in the toxic body. Cleansing is a prerequisite to building or rebuilding, for without the ability to assimilate nutrients, it is superfluous to supply them in abundance.

If you choose to take vitamin supplements, it is wise to have a reliable means of determining just exactly what your deficiencies are and what supplements are needed. There are many ways of attempting to do this: diet questionnaires, urine, saliva and blood tests, muscle testing, ElectroDermal Screening (see chapter 12), hair analysis, iridology, live cell microscopy, etc. All of these methods have their pros and cons and limitations. Beware of individuals who might use any of these methods as a tool for promoting a line of nutritional products. Seek a practitioner with no vested interest in selling a line of nutritional products: He or she will be more objective. Seek also one who is familiar with a number of testing techniques, a truly eclectic practitioner who can choose the best approach of many for your particular needs.

Each of us is unique in our body chemistry, and therefore we have unique and individual nutrient requirements. What is optimal intake of one nutrient for one individual may create a deficiency state in another. The term "biochemical individuality" was coined many years ago by Dr. Roger Williams. This concept flies in the face of the governments' "Recommended Daily Allowances," instituted over 50 years ago by the U.S. Food and Nutrition Board, and today's RDIs. These amounts represent the absolute minimum considered necessary to ward off deficiency symptoms. Given the concept of biochemical individuality, RDA and RDI guidelines are useless.

Vitamins function with enzymes. Protein molecules, together with substances known as co-enzymes make up enzymes. The co-enzyme portion is frequently a vitamin. Vitamins and minerals act as catalysts for numerous biological reactions. Vitamins and minerals exist together and work together. Vitamin C, for example, increases absorption of iron, and the B complex of vitamins is absorbed only when combined with phosphorous.

There are two categories of vitamins: water-soluble and fat-soluble. The water-solubles are not stored in the body. The tissues absorb what they can use, and the rest, we are told, is harmlessly excreted in the urine. However, if the body is overloaded with excessive amounts of a water-soluble vitamin, a burden is placed on the organs of elimination to excrete the excess. Vitamin C and B complexes are water-soluble. Because they are not stored in the body, it is necessary to regularly replenish the supply. Frequent intake is therefore preferable to single doses of these vitamins.

The fat-solubles include vitamins A, D, E and K. They are measured in units or international units (IUs), while the water-solubles are measured in milligrams (mgs.) or micrograms (mcgs.). The fat-soluble vitamins are stored in the body and, for that reason, toxic overload is possible but only probable if one is taking massive doses over a prolonged period of time. Excessive intake, however, can certainly lead to imbalance, which can create a number of problems. The fat-solubles may be taken in single doses daily since any excess is stored rather than eliminated.

It is not within the scope of this book to cover each of the individual vitamins, although the water-solubles are discussed in the next chapter. It is advisable to become familiar with the food sources of each of the vitamins, as well as deficiency symptoms of each. There are several good reference books which supply this information. Among them are *The Nutrition Almanac* and *Prescriptions for Nutritional Healing*.

MINERALS

Minerals are nutrients that exist in the body and in food. They are found in both organic and inorganic combinations. As with vitamins, it has long been believed that all minerals must be obtained from outside sources, that the body cannot manufacture its own. While vitamins can be synthesized by living matter and minerals cannot, the findings of a French scientist, Louis Kervran, indicate that biological organisms display the ability to transmute one mineral into another within the cell. Silica, for example, can be transmuted or converted into calcium (see Kervran's *Biological Transmutations* for more information on this subject). Also, the late Dr. Carry Reams, biophysicist who developed the Biological Theory of Ionization (BTI), maintained that, given certain minerals (calcium, phosphorous, potassium and iron), the body could obtain the other essential ones from the air. So, once again, traditional thinking is being challenged in the face of new ideas and discoveries.

Vitamins are required for every biochemical activity in the body. They cannot function, however, unless minerals are present. Some minerals are part of vitamins. For example, vitamin B1 contains sulfur; B12 contains cobalt. Although only 4-5% of the body weight is mineral matter, these nutrients are critically important. All of our tissues and fluids contain minerals. Minerals help maintain water and pH balance. They assist in antibody production. Hormonal secretion of glands is dependent upon mineral stimulation. In fact, all bodily processes depend upon the action of minerals.

There are 84 known minerals, 17 of which are considered to be essential in human nutrition. If there is a shortage of just one of these, the balance of activity in the entire system can be thrown off. A deficiency of a single mineral can negatively impact the entire chain of life, rendering other nutrients ineffective and useless.

Macrominerals are those that are measured in milligrams. They are needed in substantial amounts by the body and include calcium, magnesium, phosphorous, sodium, chlorine, sulfur and potassium. The remaining minerals, needed in small, sometimes minute amounts by the body, are known as trace minerals, and most are measured in micrograms. They include iodine, selenium, chromium, copper, etc. There is another class of minerals known as heavy metals. As previously discussed, these can be harmful to the body.

Trace minerals play a crucial role in electrolyte function in the body. Electrolytes are mineral salts that dissolve in the bloodstream, forming negatively and positively charged particles called ions. They provide energy to run the body and form the basis of all physical and neurological functions. Electrolytes are needed in the maintenance and repair of all body tissues and the utilization of amino acids. They maintain "osmotic equilibrium" (balanced pressure inside and outside of cells), enabling muscles and nerves to contract and wounds to heal. They also regulate the pH of the body and are essential for the growth and development of the bones and the overall maintenance of homeostasis (balance). While electrolytes are typically thought of as members of the macromineral family, it is important to know that they cannot function fully in the absence of trace minerals. Lacking certain of these, cells become oxygen deficient. The ideal electrolyte solution would therefore include trace elements.

To increase the electrical potential or life force within each cell of the body, one must first have a balance of *usable* minerals. This brings us to the topic of organic and inorganic minerals. Inorganic ones come from the earth, from soil and rock. They include the carbonates, sulfates, phosphates and oxides, all of which are poorly utilized by the body. They are not absorbed well. If they were, we could eat dirt as a direct source of our minerals! The fact is, however, that we cannot be nourished by dirt, nor can we be nourished by stones or shells that are ground up, no matter how finely. Just because we can swallow them, it doesn't mean we can utilize or assimilate them. Plants have the capacity to fully utilize inorganic minerals, however, and once they have done so, they have converted them into an *organic* form, which is usable by the human body. A mineral is organic when it has become incorporated into living tissue. We can fully utilize the organic minerals found in plants in their raw state. Minerals are rendered inorganic, however, once heat is applied in the cooking process.

A mineral in its inorganic state has to be *bound to an organic molecule* before it can pass through the intestinal wall into the bloodstream and on to the cells. This binding of an inorganic mineral to an organic molecule is known as *chelation*. When a mineral is chelated, it is altered so that it can be more readily absorbed by the body. When an inorganic mineral is chelated, it is completely surrounded by organic material, held in the "claws," so to speak, of the organic material (the word chelate means "claw"). Man has developed the ability to chelate mineral supplements (see details in the next chapter) so they will be better assimilated. The chelated mineral will target the cell, and a certain percentage of that mineral will be fully utilized. When inorganic minerals are consumed, the body cannot assimilate them and may form deposits of the unused mineral material, which leads to development of functional disorders. The human body has the capacity to chelate a small amount of inorganic minerals on its own if enough hydrochloric acid (HCl) is present. HCl is the acid that *ionizes* a mineral. Ionization is the charging of an electrically neutral substance, giving it a positive or a negative charge. Organic minerals don't need to be ionized. However, inorganic ones must first be separated from their inorganic bonds so that they can be chelated with an amino acid. Amino acids are the most commonly used chelating agents. They are the organic matter best suited for the chelation process.

According to *Senate document #264,* published in **1936**, 99% of Americans are mineral deficient. Let's look at some of the causes of this deficiency:

Insufficient HCl. Most of us have inadequate amounts of HCl in our stomachs due to excessive intake of protein and withdrawal of sodium from the tissues of the stomach to buffer excess acid in the body. Most protein foods are highly acid-forming and demand lavish secretions of HCl from the stomach. Over a period of time, the production diminishes, as the organ goes into hypo function. HCl must be present for the body to do its own chelating of inorganic minerals. In its absence, those minerals consumed will not be utilized, producing a deficiency.

High fat intake. The excessive amount of fat consumed in the SAD causes ionized minerals to bind to fats instead of amino acids, making them unavailable for absorption into the intestines.

Over-consumption of sugar and meats. Both sugar and meat are acid-forming. As previously pointed out, when the pH of the blood begins to become too acid, it must be balanced with alkaline minerals. If these are not provided from an external source, the body's storehouses are robbed, resulting in mineral depletion and deficiency.

Lack of enzymes. The SAD is enzyme poor due to over-consumption of cooked foods. Lack of enzymes in our diet makes it difficult for the body to extract minerals from foods.

Mineral deficient soils. Dr. Reams put forth the theory that all disease results from mineral deficiency. He also demonstrated how depleted our soils have become due to faulty agricultural practices, and he taught methods for accurately measuring mineral content of soil and assessing the degree of mineralization of foods coming from it. Remineralization of our soils is essential to the production of a nourishing food supply. The average fruit or vegetable of today does not have the high mineral content of its early 20th century counterpart. A great deal more of a particular food would have to be consumed today to equal the nutrient content of the same food of the early 1900s.

Even in our efforts to cleanse and rebuild the body, mineral deficiencies can occur, for minerals are rapidly depleted during detoxification and tissue rebuilding. Basically, fruits are the cleansers of the body (citrus being the most aggressive in this activity), and vegetables are the builders. Vegetables are our major source of minerals. Fresh vegetables and their juices supply the body with an abundance of organic minerals with which it can rebuild tissue. Canned, frozen and bottled vegetable juices do not have this capacity, for they have been processed with heat, which converts the organic minerals into inorganic, dead ones. Life cannot be built from death.

Dr. Paul Eck has demonstrated that not only mineral deficiencies but aberrant mineral *ratios* can adversely affect our health. The metabolic rate of an individual can be ascertained by analyzing mineral ratios measured through hair analysis and can be corrected through mineral balancing. According to Eck, restoration of health is dependent upon restoration of optimal mineral levels and ratios. Certain mineral patterns on a hair analysis reflect poor assimilation and slow metabolism, leading to a build-up of mineral deposits in the body. Random supplementation can do more harm than good according to Eck, because this can contribute to further distortion of mineral patterns. "The way people go about choosing supplements, they could do almost as well using a roulette wheel,"[6] says Eck.

Where vitamin and mineral supplements are concerned, I favor the use of super foods, nutrient dense foods that supply a wide variety of elements in their natural form. These foods include sea algae (spirulina, chlorella, dulse, kelp), land greens (barley and wheat grass), lecithin, yeast, rice bran, wheat germ, bee pollen, whey and more. A favorite of mine is mineral-rich goat whey, not only a good source of usable minerals but also a good food for beneficial gut flora.

Specific mineral deficiencies are detected in a number of ways, as previously discussed. While the traditional blood test is not generally a good tool for this, it can yield valuable information about the patient's mineral and electrolyte status when certain nonstandard interpretation parameters are applied. Such analysis has been pioneered by Lynne August, M.D. Her Health Equations program features the use of minerals, electrolytes (containing trace elements), essential fatty acids and a limited number of other nutrients used to optimize cell function. Check out her web site at www.healtheqs.com, or call 1-800-328-2818 for more information.

WATER

Water is the most abundant and important nutrient in the body. The average person can go five weeks without food but only five days without water. It is a nutrient that performs many vital functions in the body: It is a carrier for oxygen, other nutrients and metabolic waste products, helping to flush toxins out of the system; it is a chief constituent of protoplasm, 90% of the blood being made up of water; it is required for the enzymatic activity of all metabolic processes, and pure water is the primary solvent in the body, dissolving substances so that they can be assimilated or taken in by every cell. In his fine book *The Body's Many Cries for Water,* F. Batmanghelidj, M.D., notes that water is more than a solvent in the body and makes a convincing case for chronic undiagnosed dehydration as the root cause of numerous disorders, including high blood pressure, asthma, ulcers and even tumors.

Approximately 70% of the body is composed of water. This is also the percentage of our diet that ideally would be made up of high water content foods. The high water content foods are fruits, vegetables and sprouts. Consuming these gives the added advantage of helping to alkalize the system and providing fiber for the intestines. If 70% of our diet is made up of high water content foods, we can get away with less intake of exogenous water than if we were not eating such foods. However, the SAD is composed primarily of concentrated foods with little to no water content. When partaking of such a diet, large volumes of water must be consumed to replenish the nutrients in the bloodstream and to activate the kidneys so they'll be able to get rid of the excess poisonous by-products of the poorly digested foods.

Americans are not big water drinkers. In fact, we consume more soft drinks than we do water! Insufficient intake of water causes incomplete elimination — and remember: Elimination is one of the four basic elements in the C.A.R.E. model. Inadequate elimination can adversely affect the other three processes (circulation, assimilation and relaxation), resulting in a build-up of toxic accumulations.

If we are consuming a diet high in fruits, vegetables and sprouts and are therefore not particularly thirsty, then there is no need to force water into the body. Taking in too much water will eventually damage the kidneys and cause further disease. It can waterlog the tissues, impair cellular function and lower the capacity of the blood to absorb and carry oxygen. For the person on the SAD, however, thirst cannot be relied upon as a valid index of the body's need for water, as the thirst mechanism has become deranged from dietary abuse. Such a person *needs* an ample amount of exogenous water intake on a regular basis, no less than ½ oz. per pound of body weight. Soft drinks are decidedly *not* a viable option, nor is coffee, tea or pasteurized juice. Caffeine-containing beverages actually dehydrate the body further. Fresh fruits and vegetables and their juices, on the other hand, are composed largely of naturally distilled water, which will satisfy the needs of the body. Exogenous water intake should be evenly spaced throughout the day. A good rule of thumb is to drink about 4 oz. every half hour. This is preferable to guzzling down three times that amount and overworking the kidneys.

Drinking a glass of water first thing in the morning (room temperature) will provide moisture for the intestines and help keep the bowels regular. A touch of lemon in the water will help alkalize the body and support the liver.

Water leaves the stomach very rapidly — in about 5 minutes — if consumed alone. Ingesting large amounts of water with meals is to be avoided, as it will result in dilution of digestive juices.

Once we have made the basic and necessary changes in our diet, monitoring quantity of water intake becomes less of a priority. Water *quality*, however, should be an ongoing concern for all of us.

WATER QUALITY

Only 1% of the world's water is drinkable. The rest is sea water or ice. This being the case, it is critically important that we guard this precious 1% against contamination. We don't seem to be doing such a good job of this, as our own Public Health Service tells us *several million Americans* are drinking water that is potentially hazardous, contaminated with bacteria and chemicals.

Those of us on the public water system may choose to believe that our water is safe to drink because all the "bad stuff" was filtered out at the municipal water treatment plant, but this is decidedly not the case. Only suspended matter (silt, sand, etc.) can be mechanically filtered. The filtered water still contains sediment, microorganisms and dissolved chemicals. Even if the water were safe when it left the plant, there is no guarantee that it would be safe when it entered your home, for faulty pipes and soldering leaks can cause contamination. The fact of the matter is that tap water is not pure — far from it. In some cities it has been used as many as five times by other people before it reaches your home!

More than 700 different chemicals have been identified in American drinking water. The Environmental Protection Agency (EPA) tells us that our communities' water supplies are "liberally laced with asbestos, pesticides, heavy metals like lead and cadmium, arsenic, nitrates, sodium and a variety of chemicals that are known carcinogens."[7] The pollution problem has become so all pervasive that traces of DDT have been found in the ice at the North Pole! The U.S. General Accounting Office in a 3/3/82 report to the administrator of the EPA stated, "The Safe Drinking Water Act of 1974 represents the first national commitment to provide safe drinking water; yet, during fiscal year 1980, over 146,000 violations of the drinking water regulations were recorded against community water systems." (Check out www.epa.gov/enviro, an EPA web site that lists any reported violations by U.S. water suppliers in the last 10 years.)

Chemical pollution has also reached ground water (via seepage from landfills into aquifers, ruptured underground fuel oil storage tanks and septic tanks), resulting in the contamination of wells. Once contaminated, ground water can remain so for hundreds of thousands of years. The chances of contamination are good when we consider that 8 out of 10 Americans live near a toxic waste dump or source. Microorganisms linked with infectious disease can and have been transmitted through the water supply.

In many communities, water has become so polluted that it can only be made safe to drink by loading it with chlorine to kill the parasites, viruses, bacteria, algae, yeasts and molds. (Chlorine is a potent chemical used in World War II to kill *people*.) Ironically, the chlorination process itself creates carcinogens. When chlorine unites with other pollutants in the water, or even with natural organic matter such as decaying vegetation, it forms new compounds known as trihalomethanes (ThMs). ThMs consist of such deadly chemicals as chloroform, bromoform and carbon tetrachloride. Dr. Kurt Donsbach links the high incidence of kidney, bladder and urinary tract cancer in New Orleans with the fact that the water there is chlorinated in excess of government standards to guard against disease. The result is the creation of 66 new potentially carcinogenic compounds. It is also interesting that when chlorine combines with animal fat, it forms a sticky, paste-like substance that adheres to arterial walls. ThMs are a known causative agent in atherosclerosis, as are cadmium and fluoride, also found in tap water. Studies have shown a link between chlorination and increased incidences of colon and rectal cancer, as well as bladder cancer.[8]

"Dioxin, a toxic by-product of chlorine, has been found to be 300,000 times more potent as a carcinogen than DDT."[9] Plastics are a major source of dioxins, which accumulate in the fatty tissues and, because they mimic estrogen, they disrupt hormone function. Chlorine contamination from water supplies, the paper industry and household cleaning products, has become so widespread that virtually all humans have detectable levels of dioxin in their blood. Dioxin has been linked with many health problems, including depressed immunity, endometriosis, diabetes, neurotoxicity, birth defects, decreased fertility and reproductive dysfunction in both sexes.

Some people believe that boiling water will make it safe to drink. This is not so, for boiling may actually concentrate some contaminants such as fluorides. If you must drink polluted water, however, boil it for at least ten minutes. This will at least kill some of the bacteria. It will not, however, remove the inorganic minerals nor the dissolved solids and many of the chemicals.

If boiling water doesn't purify it, where can we turn for pure water — to rain water, to bottled water? When rain falls through the air, it picks up the bacteria, dust, smoke, chemicals and minerals there, so the water is no longer pure by the time it reaches earth. As far as bottled water is concerned, the standards for it are basically the same as for municipal water systems. In fact, some bottled water has been found to actually come straight from the tap!

Perhaps our best pure water source is the water found in organic fruits and vegetables. It is distilled by nature. The distilling process turns water into vapor and, through condensation, back again into pure water. Electric distillers do the same thing. Another effective way to purify water is through Reverse Osmosis (RO). Here contaminates are removed when water is forced through a semi-permeable membrane. Most RO systems also employ a pre-filter to trap sediment and a carbon filter to remove chlorine, some metals and pesticides. Carbon filters used alone are ineffective in ridding water of numerous other pollutants, including parasites and bacteria. Both distillation and RO purification remove nutritive minerals along with contaminants. There is no known way to remove just the pollutants and leave the minerals.

Demineralized water (RO and distilled) is hungry water that will aggressively leach chemicals such as vinyl chloride out of plastic jugs. Purified water therefore should always be stored in glass containers, unless minerals have been added back to the water right after treatment. I've come to believe that it is necessary to do just that, to add minerals back (using a liquid mineral supplement) to purified water for our health's sake. Minerals found in water are far better assimilated by the body than those found in food. To rely totally on food as a source of minerals is unwise, especially in view of the mineral depletion of the soils.

Studies have repeatedly shown that people drinking "hard" water (high in calcium carbonate) have a lower incidence of heart disease than those drinking soft water. Such studies are using tap water, which is universally polluted and should never be ingested. If you must drink such water, however, you are better off with hard than soft, for the minerals in it will prevent absorption of the heavy metals that are, no doubt, also present and can lead to heart disease and other ailments.

Purity has typically been the single factor used to judge water quality, and by this parameter alone, we might view distilled water as superior. However, two other parameters need to be considered when evaluating the "biological compatibility" of water. These parameters were established by noted European hydrologists, physicists and doctors in over 20 years of research. Important findings were made by the late Professor Luis Vincent while serving as chief hydrologist in France. Based on his work, three parameters for biological compatibility were identified: resistivity (purity), pH (acidity/alkalinity) and RH2 (oxidation/reduction, a measurement of electrons). An instrument known as the Bioelectronic Vincent (BEV) was designed to test fluids (blood, urine and saliva, as well as water) according to these parameters. Ideal values were established, and it was found by Vincent and his colleague, the late German doctor, Franz Morrell, that only very few naturally-occurring waters on the planet met the criteria for biological compatibility. They had originally believed that no treated water could meet these standards (pH 5.3-6.8 and RH2 between 25 and 29, as well as extremely high R, purity). However, in 1984, Dr. Morrell endorsed the RO process as capable of meeting all three standards of biological compatibility. Vincent's BEV work forms the basis of today's Biological Terrain Assessment (BTA).

While not all RO units meet Vincent's standards, the better ones do, and the RO process itself would seem to produce a water of higher vitality than that produced through the distillation process which yields water that has often been described as "dead."

No discussion of water quality would be complete without mentioning a major pollutant which permeates an alarming percentage of our water supply:

FLUORIDE

Sodium fluoride and sodium silico fluoride are by-products of the aluminum and phosphate fertilizer industries. In 1937, Dr. Gerald Fox of the Mellon Institute began to suggest publicly that fluoride prevented tooth decay. Just coincidentally, the Mellon Institute was associated with the Aluminum Company of America (ALCOA). The sale of fluoride to cities for use in their water systems and to manufacturers of toothpaste, mouthwash, etc. presents a lucrative outlet for an otherwise useless, undesirable, *toxic waste.*

One of the most outspoken and fluent opponents of water fluoridation is Dr. John Yiamouyiannis, author of *Fluoride The Aging Factor.* Dr. Yiamouyiannis holds a Ph.D. in biochemistry and is former editor at Chemical Abstracts Service, the world's largest chemical information center. Serving in that position, he was able to gather much information on fluoride. Dr. Yiamouyiannis opens his book by taking us to a village in Turkey where the residents age prematurely, exhibiting wrinkles and brittle bones, etc. in their 30s, with many not even living to age 50. Their condition is attributed to the 5.4 parts per million (ppm) of natural fluoride found in their drinking water. Where this same fluoride level is found in the water in parts of India, the same kind of age-accelerating effects are noted. (A lower amount of naturally-occurring fluoride does not seem to produce such results, particularly when it is found in hard water, which also contains high levels of calcium. Since calcium is the neutralizer for fluoride poisoning, fluoride brings its own antidote.) It is interesting to note, with this in mind, that one of the original studies supporting the use of sodium fluoride to reduce tooth decay was done in the town of Hereford, Texas in the 1940s, where the residents' low incidence of dental caries was attributed to the relatively high content of natural fluorine in the water. This study was sponsored by *the Aluminum Trust!* It was followed by a study in New York involving a large number of school children in two nearby communities, Kingston and Newburgh. It was reported — by the Aluminum Trust — that the Newburgh kids, drinking fluoridated water had 60% fewer cavities than their Kingston counterparts who drank non-fluoridated water. Follow-up studies by objective sources have not upheld these results, however. It has been found that the decay rate has declined more in the non-fluoridated city of Newburgh in the last 30+ years. It seems, as other evidence supports, that the use of fluoride only *delays* the formation of cavities. And, while tooth decay rates are now declining in fluoridated areas, they are likewise dropping at the same rate in non-fluoridated areas.

Dr. Yiamouyiannis, along with the late Dr. Dean Burk, published epidemiological studies in the mid-1970s showing that cancer rates in fluoridated areas were higher than in non-fluoridated ones. Based on these findings, Congress ordered a 10-year study by the National Toxicology Program of the EPA in 1977. By 1989, their research was completed but not yet published, as it awaited a "peer review." Their unreleased report indicated that bone cancer and bone tumors occurred in laboratory test animals from fluoride. Proctor and Gamble performed a study with similar findings.

In 1986-87, the National Institute of Dental Research gathered data on nearly 40,000 school children from 84 geographical areas. Under the Freedom of Information Act, Yiamouyiannis obtained their data, analyzed it and found no differences in the percentage of decay-free children in the fluoridated and non-fluoridated groups and no significant differences between decay rates of the two groups.

Sodium fluoride, added to drinking water, is entirely different from naturally-occurring calcium fluoride found in oats, sunflower seeds, mackerel, raw milk, cheese, garlic, beet tops, green, leafy vegetables, almonds, sea water and hard water. Inorganic sodium fluoride is an instant poison. Fluoride is listed in the 24th edition of the *U.S. Dispensary* as a known poison used to kill weeds and rodents. So — it is rat poison with which we are treating our cities' water supplies in the name of preventing tooth decay on the authority of the aluminum interests ... Makes about as much sense as disposing of nuclear waste in our food supply!!

Actually, the most common forms of fluoride added to drinking water today are the silicofluorides (SiF), which include fluorosilicates and fluorosilicic acid (FSA), a by-product of the phosphate fertilizer industry. FSA, along with other toxins, is collected in air pollution scrubbers. These other toxins include heavy metals, along with other industrial contaminants, and constitute about 75% of the actual substance used to fluoridate water supplies. The other 25% is FSA.

Dartsmouth researchers found in a study published in 1999 in *The International Journal of Environmental Studies* that lead levels in children's blood were significantly higher in Massachusetts communities where the water was fluoridated with SiF than in towns where water was treated with sodium fluoride or not fluoridated at all. Fluoride increases not only lead but also aluminum levels. Fluoridated water used in conjunction with aluminum cookware is therefore a deadly combination.

Fluorine is not a mineral. It is a nonmetallic gaseous element much like chlorine. It is given off in waste gases from aluminum factories. Over the last 50 years, industries have released 725,000,000 tons of fluoride gases and particulates into the atmosphere. It has been found that the herbivorous animals in the vicinity of these fluoride-emitting factories exhibit signs of fluorosis (fluoride poisoning) after eating vegetation that has absorbed the fluorine through the air. Fluorides are formed when the fluorine ion unites with metals.

The U.S. Pharmacopoeia lists some of the side-effects that can result from the daily ingestion of the amount of fluoride found in 1-2 pints of artificially fluoridated water:

   black tarry stools
   bloody vomit
   faintness
   nausea and vomiting
   shallow breathing
   stomach cramps or pain
   tremors
   unusual excitement
   unusual increase in saliva
   watery eyes
   weakness
   constipation
   loss of appetite
   pain and aching of bones
   skin rash
   sores in the mouth and on the lips
   stiffness
   weight loss
   white, brown or black discoloration of teeth

The discoloration of teeth is known as "mottling" and is a common result of fluorosis.

Dr. Leo Spira, who conducted experiments with fluoride on rats for four years, found that it interferes with the proper utilization of B vitamins, damages the thyroid gland and kidneys and causes the heart muscle to become flabby and degenerate. Not only can fluoride lower thyroid activity, it was at one time used medically to depress the activity of the thyroid gland, according to the *Merck Index.*(10)

Teeth and bone are the most fluoride-sensitive tissues in the body. A retention of 2 mg. of fluoride per day is calculated to result in skeletal fluorosis in 40 years for the average individual. Fluorosis of the skeleton in its clinical phases produces moderate to severe arthritic symptoms.

Dr. Yiamouyiannis reports that fluoride also interferes with enzyme activity by reforming hydrogen bonds. It accelerates the breakdown of collagen (the major structural component of skin, ligaments, tendons, cartilage, bone and teeth). This can result in the mineralization of tissues that should not be mineralized and the demineralization of tissues that should remain mineralized. Mineralization has a hardening effect, and demineralization has a softening effect. So, soft teeth and bones can be the net result of excessive fluoride intake, regardless of any immediate dental benefits that may be claimed. Dr. Spira lists otosclerosis of the ears (deafness) and sclerosis of the arteries among the symptoms of fluorosis. Sclerosis is hardening, mineralization. Dr. Spira also lists bone cancer as a consequence of fluorosis. Dr. Dean Burk, former chief biochemist at the National Cancer Institute, stated long ago that "more than 50,000 Americans a year are dying of cancer caused by fluoridated drinking water," and added that "any institution who supports fluoridation is guilty of mass murder."

Dr. Yiamouyiannis states that fluoride interferes with the use of oxygen in the body — It depresses the synthesis of ATP. With depression of ATP production, we don't have fuel to run the electrical generators (sodium/potassium pump) in the body, and the stage is set for development of degenerative disease.

The June 1960 edition of *The Herald of Health* quoted the then Medical Director of Marin County, California as saying, "Fluoride is toxic to a segment of the population, the older age group, in that it interferes with calcium metabolism. It causes osteoporosis in the older age group; it has been known to cause tetany-form convulsions." It stands to reason that fluoride ingestion can lead to osteoporosis, given the disruption of the collagen-forming mechanism it causes. And yet, some medical doctors today are actually treating osteoporosis with fluoride!

Fluoride, as uranium hexafluoride, was actually the key chemical used in atomic bomb production. As such, its dangers were well-known to government officials who kept the information classified during and after World War II. During the Cold War period, millions of tons of fluoride were used to manufacture high-grade uranium and plutonium for nuclear weapons. It was fluoride poisoning resulting from the atomic weapons program, rather than radiation damage caused by it, that actually formed the basis of the first lawsuits against that program.

Over twenty years ago, the California State Department of Agriculture outlawed the fluoridation of milk and ordered fluoride removed from fertilizers *because of its highly poisonous effect on plant life* — and yet we put it in our water!? Fluoride was outlawed in ten European countries as of 1984.(11) Today, less than 2% of the European population have fluoridated water supplies.

The amount of fluoride used in water fluoridation is 1 ppm. It is not possible, however, to maintain a fixed dosage, and the mixture may deviate lower or higher. Even at 1 ppm, fluoride use has been linked with birth defects, Mongolism, heart and kidney diseases, allergies and cancer. Dr. Sheila Gibson from the University of Glasgow showed that fluoride, at levels comparable to those found in the blood of people living in fluoridated areas, decreased the migration rate of human white blood cells. This is highly significant, for it means the immune response is seriously depressed.

Fluoride is highly injurious to both water mains and water supplies, for it attacks almost everything and eats through metal materials. Analysis of water mains in fluoridated cities has shown concentrations as high as 8000 ppm (Concord, Massachusetts, 1/29/59, as per Standard Laboratories). Some cities have eliminated fluoridation strictly on the basis of increased cost of repair of water mains. In the last decade, over 45 U.S. cities have rejected fluoridation.

Chronic fluoride poisoning affects the section of the brain concerned with volition and the will to resist. Experiments on rats have shown marked deterioration in mental alertness, accompanied by a state of "passive bewilderment." Zoo keepers and animal trainers use sodium fluoride on their animals to pacify them. Fighting bulls given 1 ppm became so docile they refused to charge. Does this tell us something about the political ramifications of water fluoridation??

In the 1980s, 108 million Americans were drinking fluoridated water, and 25% of households used fluoridated toothpaste or other fluoridated products. Today, most certainly the majority of households use such products, for it is no longer possible to buy a major brand of toothpaste that is not fluoridated. About 60% of the American population now drinks fluoridated water. It has become widespread practice to launch fluoride campaigns in public schools, and routine dental checkups invariably include fluoride treatments for children.

"Effects of Chronic Exposure to Low Level Pollutants" (a report prepared by the Library of Congress' Congressional Research Service for the U.S. House Subcommittee on the Environment and the Atmosphere) lists fluoride (along with chlorines, asbestos, nickel and mercury) as a pollutant that is dangerous due to its adverse effect on the central nervous system and the increased risk of cancer, heart disease and genetic mutations it poses. According to chemistry indexes, sodium fluoride is more toxic than lead and only a little less toxic than arsenic. Interestingly, "The Center for Disease Control in the U.S. and the British Ministry of Health both admit that no credible study has shown fluoride to be of any benefit whatsoever."[12]

Word has gotten out that fluoride is a toxic drug. Fluoridated toothpastes in the U.S. are now required by the FDA to have warning labels. There is enough fluoride in a tube of toothpaste to kill a small child. In fact, on 1/29/79, a New York State Supreme Court jury awarded $750,000 to the parents of a three-year old boy who was administered a lethal dose of fluoride during a routine treatment at a dental clinic. The hygienist had neglected to tell him not to swallow the solution. This was not an isolated incident. On more than one occasion lately, scientists who previously supported fluoridation, have spoken openly against it.[13] Dr. Robert Carton, EPA scientist for 20 years, describes fluoridation as "the greatest case of scientific fraud of this century, if not all time."

Fluoride also poses a health hazard in the form of hexafluoride (HF) used in lead-free gasoline to achieve high octane ratings. This substance, though more toxic than lead, now replaces it in automotive exhaust.

According to information found at http://www.rvi.net/~fluoride/index.htm, "The electric power industry uses sulfur hexafluoride (SF6) to insulate high voltage lines, circuit breakers and other equipment in electricity transmission and distribution. The gas escapes through electrical equipment seals and is released when equipment is damaged. Older circuit breakers tend to leak the gas at a faster rate than newer equipment."

We can see from the information presented here that there are many sources of fluoride contamination in our environment today.

Even if your water is not fluoridated, chances are better than good that it is polluted to a dangerous level whether it comes from the municipal plant or your own well. In view of the hazard posed by fluoride and the hundreds of other toxins lacing our water supply, it is vitally important that we purify our water — preferably with an RO unit. It is further advised that minerals be restored to the newly purified water through the addition of a liquid supplement. Odorless, tasteless products are available that will do nicely for this purpose. It is advisable to avoid drinking water in restaurants and from water fountains. Carry your own remineralized pure water with you, and drink an ample amount of it daily, especially if your intake of fruits and vegetables is low.

CHAPTER 11

Some Specific Nutrients
(Calcium, B and C Vitamins)

*"One cannot think well, love well, sleep well,
if one has not dined well."*
Virginia Woolf

I have chosen in this chapter to discuss calcium and vitamins B and C complexes, to the exclusion of the many other nutrients, due to their popularity — and the many misconceptions regarding them.

CALCIUM

The American public has developed a calcium consciousness in recent years, one that is permeated with a great deal of misinformation. Once again we have a case of the erroneous "more is better" philosophy rearing its head. We have allowed ourselves to be convinced through simplistic reasoning and the food industry's advertising campaigns that inadequate calcium consumption is the cause of calcium deficiency and the consequent development of such degenerative diseases as osteoporosis. Believing this, conscientious "health conscious" Americans are now increasing their intake of the popular calcium rich foods — namely dairy products. My aim in this section is to address some of the popular misconceptions regarding reasons for calcium deficiency and to identify desirable food sources of this important mineral. Dr. Carey Reams believed calcium to be *the* most important of all the minerals. He stated that plants, animals and humans need more it by weight and volume than any other mineral. Dr. Reams observed that there are over 250,000 different kinds and 7 groups of calcium, one of which is toxic to all life. The body, he maintained, needs some of the other six every day. Calcium is the most abundant mineral in the body. Deficiency symptoms include:

- nervous tension
- tetany
- bone malformation (rickets, osteomalacia)
- osteoporosis
- joint pain
- muscle cramps and spasms
- heart palpitation
- slow pulse
- insomnia
- tooth decay
- impaired growth
- decreased glandular function
- excessive irritability of nerves and muscles

No one would argue that the increased incidence of osteoporosis would be indicative of a widespread calcium deficiency. What is arguable, however, is the contention that this deficiency is due to inadequate intake of calcium-rich foods. Indications are that it is not inadequate intake, but rather *decreased availability* of the mineral, which is the prime cause of most deficiency conditions. Contrary to popular belief, dairy products are not the best source of calcium. The chart below (information from the U.S. Department of Agriculture and the Japan Nutritionist Association) gives the calcium content of various foods per 100 grams, expressed in milligrams:

DAIRY FOODS:

Cow's milk	118
Goat's milk	120
Cheese, various	250

VEGETABLES:

Turnip greens	130
Kale	179
Mustard greens	183
Parsley	200
Leaf-beet	100
Spinach	93-98
Watercress	90
Collard greens	203

BEANS AND BEAN PRODUCTS:

Kidney beans	130
Broad beans	100
Soybeans	130
Tofu (soybean curd)	128
Natto (fermented soybeans)	92-103

*SEAWEEDS (Sea Vegetables):

Kombu	800
Hijiki	1,400
Wakame	1,300
Arame	1,170
Agar-agar	400

*SEEDS AND NUTS:

Sesame seeds	1,160
Sunflower seeds	140
Sweet almonds	282
Brazil nuts	186
Hazel nuts	209

(*an average serving is 1/2 or less of the amount listed)

Also rich in calcium are many fish and seafoods, especially sardines and shellfish. Shellfish are not a particularly good choice, however, as they filter bacteria, viruses and toxic substances out of polluted waters and concentrate them in their flesh. Please note that the seaweeds or sea vegetables, which are a mainstay in the macrobiotic approach to eating, are by far the richest source of calcium. These sea vegetables are also exceedingly rich in other minerals and for this reason are a helpful addition to the mineral-poor SAD. Dulse and kelp are two sea vegetables that are not listed. They can be purchased in granulated form and make an excellent condiment. They're actually very low in sodium but have a salty taste resulting from the abundance of other minerals. Kelp contains 1,093 mg. of calcium per 100 grams — dulse 567. The latter is the one seaweed that can be eaten directly out of the package without having to be soaked in water first. It makes a tasty mineral-rich snack.

Notice that sesame seeds are very high in calcium. So, too, is tahini or sesame butter (like peanut butter, only made from sesame seeds). This nutritious food makes a good snack. It should not, however, be spread on bread, as this makes for a poor food combination (the protein of the seed + the starch of the bread). Try it on celery. Notice, too, from the chart that the green, leafy vegetables are as rich or richer than milk in calcium. It is important that we consume these vegetables or their juices in their raw state so that we ingest the calcium in its usable, organic form. Fresh raw vegetable juice is a rich source of readily available minerals, including calcium. Juicing is a practice that will eliminate the vegetable fiber, providing us with a rich source of vitamins and minerals in the juice. Juicing one pound of vegetables is equivalent to eating 15 pounds as far as nutritive value is concerned. A large glass of freshly squeezed juice has more food value than all three of the day's meals combined. When we eat a vegetable, 90% or more of its nutrients are eliminated in the fiber as it passes through the body. When we drink the juice of that same vegetable, however, we get 100% of the food value, and we get it immediately, as the nutrients from fresh juices are available to the body in minutes. Hydraulic press juicers maintain more of the nutrients from the food than do the centrifugal force variety but are more costly. A good centrifugal force juicer with pulp ejector can be very effective. No kitchen should be without a juicer of some sort. It is more important than your cooking utensils.

Getting back to the subject of calcium, I highly recommend a high intake of green, leafy vegetables (and their juices) as a superior source of calcium. Juiced carrots are a great source of usable calcium. Remember: The minerals (including calcium) from plants are organic and therefore can be fully utilized by the body. Once we have cooked the plant, however, or pasteurized its juice, we not only reduce the mineral content but convert the remaining minerals to an inorganic form, which the body cannot assimilate and which will very likely end up as calcium deposits somewhere in the body and cause distress.

In support of the notion that it is decreased availability of calcium, not inadequate intake of it, that is the primary causative factor in deficiency of the mineral, consider some of these reasons for the poor assimilation:

(1) **INADEQUATE INTAKE OF VITAMIN D, MAGNESIUM, ES-SENTIAL FATTY ACIDS (EFAs) AND SILICA.** In order for the body to utilize calcium, it must have a sufficient quantity of vitamin D. This can be acquired either by ingestion or through exposure to the sun. The sun's ultraviolet rays activate a form of cholesterol in the skin, converting it to vitamin D. The type of vitamin D found in pasteurized milk is vitamin D2, calciferol, a synthetic form. In milk, this form of vitamin D binds with magnesium and carries it out of the body.

Magnesium is essential to many body functions. The balance between it and calcium is especially important. If calcium consumption is increased, magnesium consumption must also be increased. The ideal ratio of calcium to magnesium is a matter of some contention. For years it was thought that we should consume twice as much calcium as magnesium, and all mineral supplements were formulated using this ratio. Most still are. In recent years, however, the efficacy of this ratio has been seriously questioned — by Dr. Guy Abraham, M.D., for one. He maintains that the optimal calcium/magnesium ratio is just the opposite of what we've thought — 2 parts magnesium to 1 part calcium. He points out that man evolved on a diet high in magnesium (found primarily in fresh green vegetables, whole grains, seeds and nuts) and low in calcium. To increase calcium intake without increasing magnesium consumption (as we're doing today), Dr. Abraham claims, results in premature aging through calcification of soft tissue. He points out that the body can store calcium but not magnesium. Therefore, if too much calcium and too little magnesium are consumed, calcium deposits can build up in the body. Too much calcium in the cells will calcify the mitochondria, the power source of the cell, and suppress ATP production, Dr. Abraham states.

Magnesium, he tells us, keeps calcium in solution and prevents formation of deposits in arteries and joints. The U.S. now has the highest RDA for calcium in the world. It was raised from 400 mg. daily to 800 mg. after World War II due to the influence of a medical doctor named Sherman who was appointed to set up the RDA for calcium. Dr. Abraham tells us *he had a big grant from the dairy council.*(1) While the RDA for calcium went up, the RDA for magnesium *dropped* from 400 to 300 mg., with further drops anticipated. In 1989, the RDA for calcium for 18-24 year olds was raised to 1200 mg. So, our RDA for calcium is the highest in the world, while that for magnesium is the lowest. This being the case, if Dr. Abraham is correct about ideal ratio of calcium to magnesium, we are creating more of a problem rather than solving an existing one, by adhering to government RDA standards and following their nutritional advice. If you take mineral supplements, deciding on the correct calcium/magnesium ratio can create a dilemma under the circumstances. It might therefore be the better part of wisdom to look to food sources for these minerals, with an emphasis on fresh juices and land and sea vegetables. We can count on nature to know and provide the proper ratio.

EFA deficiencies can prevent assimilation of calcium, for these fatty acids combine with vitamin D to make calcium available to the tissues. The widespread deficiency of certain EFAs and the causes for it have already been touched upon.

Lastly, the trace mineral silica (found largely in plant fiber; most abundantly in horsetail and shavegrass herbs) appears to work with calcium to make strong bones. It has been found, in fact, that broken bones do not knit when there are high amounts of calcium but little or no silica. They heal well with an abundance of silica and the proper calcium in the diet. The French scientists tell us that the body can convert or transmute silica into calcium.(2)

(2)   **INTERFERENCE FROM CERTAIN DRUGS.** The ingestion of aluminum-containing antacids causes an increase in calcium excretion from the body. TUMS is advertised as an excellent source of calcium. The type of calcium (carbonate) it provides, however, reduces stomach acid, and, since calcium cannot be assimilated without sufficient HCl, the calcium in the TUMS is not usable by the body. Corticosteroids (cortisone), diuretics and the anticoagulant heparin also interfere with calcium absorption.

(3)   **LACK OF EXERCISE.** Being confined to bed rest following an illness results in depletion of calcium from the bones and nitrogen from the muscle tissues. For this reason, physical activity is encouraged as soon as possible during recovery.

(4)   **LACK OF HCl.** Most of us lack HCl due, in part, to overconsumption of protein, requiring an acid secretion for digestion. HCl deficiency also results from sodium leaching from the stomach to buffer excess food acids. Those will blood type A tend to be especially low in HCl, needed to assimilate calcium.

(5)   **TOO MUCH DIETARY FAT.** Excess fat combines with calcium to form insoluble calcium soaps, which cannot be assimilated.

(6)   **TOO MUCH PHOSPHORUS.** A ratio of 2.5 parts calcium to 1 part phosphorus in the bones is maintained by the healthy body. Meat is very high in phosphorus; so are soft drinks, which contain phosphoric acid (to keep the bubbles from going flat). Over-consumption of both of these creates an excess intake of phosphorus and throws off the calcium/phosphorus ratio. Phosphoric acid in sodas binds with magnesium and pulls both minerals out of the body.

(7)   **FLUOROSIS.** Fluoride poisoning, as previously discussed, disrupts collagen formation, impairing calcium metabolism.

(8)   **ELECTROMAGNETIC POLLUTION.** Discussed fully in chapter 8, we find that one adverse effect of high amplitude "extremely low frequency" fields, such as found near high tension lines, is interference with calcium metabolism.

(9)   **INORGANIC OXALIC ACID CONSUMPTION.** The green, leafy vegetables (spinach, Swiss chard, French sorrel, turnip and mustard greens, kale, collards) contain oxalic acid, which, in its raw, organic state, is beneficial to the body. It stimulates peristalsis. Oxalic acid combines with calcium in the body. If both are organic, we have a workable combination, with the oxalic acid assisting in the digestion of the calcium. However, when the oxalic acid has become inorganic as a result of cooking or processing of foods that contain it, then it forms an interlocking bond with any calcium ingested at the same meal and destroys the nutritive value of both. The net result is serious calcium deficiency. When oxalic acid is converted to an inorganic acid, it often results in the creation of oxalic acid crystals in the kidneys. Calcium oxalate is a major component of kidney stones.

(10)   **OVER-CONSUMPTION OF PHYTIC ACID.** Phytic acid is an organic acid found in the outer husks of grains. When the whole grain is consumed, there is little risk of consuming too much phytic acid. However, when the bran and germ are removed from the grain and consumed separately in large amounts, we can have problems, for calcium tends to bind with the phytic acid and form an insoluble complex not usable by the body. Soaking grains overnight in water (to which vitamin C powder is added to acidify it and counteract toxins) helps eliminate the phytic acid.

(11)   **CONSUMPTION OF PASTEURIZED PRODUCTS.** The pasteurization process is discussed more fully later in this chapter. The point has already been made — and bears repeating — that the heat used in the pasteurization process converts organic into inorganic minerals, which are not well assimilated. Calcium from pasteurized milk, being inorganic, is not fully assimilable by the body.

(12)   **EXCESS USE OF ALCOHOL, TOBACCO, SUGAR.** Use of these stimulants increases the need for calcium to neutralize the acidity that they create in the system.

(13)   **EXCESS PROTEIN CONSUMPTION.** Like the above mentioned items, over-consumption of protein creates an acid condition in the body. Calcium, being an alkaline mineral, is pulled from the body's own tissues to balance pH if a usable form of the mineral is not supplied in the diet. It is entirely possible to have the cells starved for calcium while heavy calcium deposits build up outside of them.

(14)   **INSUFFICIENT PROTEIN CONSUMPTION.** While too much protein can cause a calcium deficiency, so can too little protein. According to Dr. Lynne August (*Health Equations Newsletter,* Fall 1998), "Minerals are deposited in a protein matrix within the bone. If there is insufficient dietary protein, the body cannot maintain this protein matrix."

(15)   **EXCESSIVE SALT INTAKE.** Table salt is an inorganic form of sodium. The more table salt you take in, the more calcium you excrete. Table salt should be strictly avoided and replaced with an unprocessed salt. I recommend Celtic sea salt, available from the Grain and Salt Society (1-800-TOP SALT)

(16)   **OROTIC ACID DEFICIENCY.** Inability of the body to synthesize this element of the B complex will adversely affect calcium utilization, for orotic acid pulls calcium into the bones. If our livers aren't able to produce orotic acid, instead of getting into the bones, calcium is deposited in soft tissues.

(17)   **TRACE MINERAL DEFICIENCY.** Silica, one trace mineral, has already been discussed. Not only silica, however, but all of the trace minerals are vitally important for calcium absorption, for lacking them, the body doesn't produce enough digestive acids or enzymes, which causes poor assimilation of calcium and other minerals. A significant study in the *Journal of Nutrition* (1994;124: 1060-1064) showed that the addition of trace minerals alone (zinc, copper and manganese) to the diet slows bone loss, and when these trace minerals are taken along with a calcium citrate, bone loss is reversed and bone density increased in post menopausal women.

It is not difficult to get calcium into the stomach and blood circulation, but it is not that easy to get to the cellular level, where we quite literally live or die.

I have already mentioned that the RDA went up to 800 mg. daily after World War II (1200 for teenagers). Many nutritionists recommend even more, a daily intake of between 1000 and 1500 mg. Since the SAD typically contains only 450-500 mg. of calcium, it is tempting to conclude that we are not taking in enough. Dr. Samuel West tells us, however, that of 800 mg. of calcium consumed daily, 700 are excreted in the feces, and that portion of the remaining 100 that is not stored in the bones is eventually excreted in the urine.(3)   Our actual calcium requirements therefore appear to be quite low.

Excess calcium is picked up by the blood and deposited in soft tissues. The excessive intake of calcium prevents phosphate absorption by forming insoluble phosphate products. This draining of phosphorus out of the body interferes with ATP production (and therefore the production of electrical energy), according to Dr. West.(4)

Osteoporosis is a condition of too little bone mass. The bones in an osteoporosis victim are brittle, weak and very susceptible to fracture. Usually the disease is not diagnosed until a person falls down, breaks a bone, and the x-ray reveals a bone mass that looks like Swiss cheese. Osteoporosis affects 15 million Americans and is present today in women as young as 25 years of age. Women need more calcium than do men and are eight times more likely to develop osteoporosis than men. Men are not exempt, however. We have all seen the stooped over little old man whose spine is crooked because the vertebrae have collapsed due to osteoporosis.

Ninety-nine percent of the body's calcium is stored in the bones and teeth. The other 1% is in the blood for use in such vital functions as contraction of heart muscles, clotting of blood and beating of the heart. To maintain life, the body will see to it that a sufficient blood level of calcium is maintained and will steal from the bones and teeth, if necessary, to do so. For this reason, blood tests do not provide reliable measures of calcium levels in the body. The serum calcium level is not indicative of how much calcium there is in the cell system. We may have a normal level of calcium in the blood and still have bones that look like Swiss cheese.

Pasteurized dairy products are undesirable for the osteoporosis patient for reasons discussed in the next section. Commercial dairy products do not prevent osteoporosis. If they did, we should have a very low incidence of it, for we consume more dairy products than any other country in the world — 300 pounds per person per year! And yet our incidence of the disease is very high. In fact, *the highest incidence of osteoporosis occurs in countries where dairy products and calcium supplements are consumed in the greatest quantity, and the lowest incidence is in countries where the least amount of these products is consumed.*

MILK

As you may have gathered by now, I do not consider milk to be an acceptable source of calcium — at least not pasteurized, homogenized cow's milk. While raw milk provides us with a source of organic calcium, when the milk is heated to 115° the soluble calcium becomes insoluble so the body can't digest it. As Dr. Norman Walker long ago observed, temperatures from 190°- 230° are required to kill such pathogenic organisms as typhoid, bacilli coli, tuberculosis and undulant fever. In the pasteurization process, however, temperatures between 145° and 170° are used.(5) True: This process does kill some harmful bacteria, but it also destroys beneficial bacteria whose job it is to keep the putrefactive bacteria in check. Ironically then, pasteurization destroys the germicidal properties of milk. It also destroys vitamins, minerals and enzymes (including phosphatase, which is necessary for the assimilation of calcium). It changes the chemical structure of the protein and renders it and the minerals less digestible and assimilable. "Yes, but it kills bad germs," your conditioning may be asserting. Consider this: Within *24-48 hours after pasteurization, the amount of bacteria in the milk doubles!*(6) Of course, it is of utmost importance that milk be produced and handled under sanitary conditions, but "pasteurized" does not mean the same as "clean;" it means heated. Pasteurized milk can be unclean, and the process can actually serve to mask the spoilage. Pasteurization was initiated in 1895. As its use became more widespread, the health of the nation declined. Pasteurized, homogenized cow's milk is extremely mucus-forming and very constipating. Even baby cows cannot tolerate it. Studies have shown that calves fed such milk died in 30 days!(7) It is interesting, too, that juvenile delinquency is highly correlated with high intake of pasteurized cow's milk.(8)

So, what are the alternatives to drinking pasteurized, homogenized milk? There are two: Drink raw milk, or don't drink milk. If you are over 4 years old, the latter is not a bad alternative. We are the only animal that continues to drink milk after we have been weaned. There are two elements in milk that have to be broken down — lactose and casein. The breakdown of lactose requires the presence of the enzyme lactase, which is not present in 98% of the adult population, thus the prevalence of "lactose intolerance." Casein is the protein component in milk. Its breakdown requires the presence of the enzyme rennin which is gone in most of us by age 3 or 4. The casein content of cow's milk is *300 times higher than in mother's milk*. Casein is a tenacious adhesive glue used to glue wood together. Mucus production is a byproduct of the bacterial decomposition of casein in the body. So, there is ample reason to give up milk if you are an adult.

The other option is to use raw milk and raw milk products. In most states it is illegal to buy and sell raw milk, however. Few states legally deal in "medically certified raw milk," milk that is certified to have been produced under sanitary conditions. Even in states where raw milk cannot be legally obtained, it is often possible to legally purchase raw milk products, such as cheese and butter, through health food stores.

Apart from the issue of raw vs. pasteurized, consider the animals from which the milk comes. If you must drink the milk of another species, I recommend goat's milk as superior to cow's. It is easier to digest (20 minutes vs. 2-3 hours) and assimilate, and it is closer in chemical composition to human milk than any other known milk. The baby goat weighs 6-10 lbs., about the same as a human infant. The newborn calf, on the other hand, is a tremendously large animal in comparison, weighing approximately 65 lbs. It is not surprising that the chemical composition of the milk of such an animal is vastly different from human milk. The fat globules in cow's milk are too large for the human body to process, while goat's milk is naturally homogenized. Drinking goat's milk might seem exotic to us, but actually most of the world's population (3/5) drinks it. The goat is the healthiest domestic animal known, and her milk contains more vitamins than any other food on the planet. Goat's milk is excellent for stomach conditions and kidney disturbances. Dr. Bernard Jensen recommends its use for babies and invalids in such conditions as tuberculosis, constipation, malnutrition, rickets, anemia, nervousness, weight loss, stomach ulcers and asthma. He emphasizes its germicidal effect and its ability to clear catarrhal conditions due to a high fluorine content.(9) The benefits spoken of here apply only to RAW goat's milk. The pasteurized variety is to be avoided. While goat's milk is naturally homogenized, the homogenization of cow's milk is a process devised by man about which I have as much concern as pasteurization.

HOMOGENIZATION

Homogenizing milk changes the structure of its fat molecules. It breaks them up into tiny particles so that they are evenly distributed. Non-homogenized cow's milk has cream floating on the top.

Research by Dr. Kurt A. Oster, a leading cardiologist (as reported in the 8/78 issue *of Acres USA),* cited homogenized milk as a major cause of heart disease in this country. The following year it was reported that Dr. Kurt Esselbacher, chairman of Harvard Medical School's Department of Medicine, drew the same conclusion, "Homogenized milk, because of its XO content (an enzyme, xanthine oxidase), is one of the major causes of heart disease in the U.S."(10)

In non-homogenized milk, XO is digested in the stomach. In homogenized milk, fat globules encase the enzyme. It therefore passes through the stomach undigested and enters the bloodstream. It has an affinity for a compound found in the artery walls, and, should it become detached from its casing of fat there, it will, via a chemical reaction, cause an abrasion in that artery wall. *The body tries to repair this abrasion with cholesterol, calcium and other minerals.*

All commercial dairy products, including skim milk and ice cream, are homogenized. The homogenization process does not improve the taste or nutritional value of milk. *All it does is prolong shelf life.*

In addition to pasteurization and homogenation, another danger of drinking commercial milk is the possible presence of rBGH.

rBGH

Recombinant Bovine Growth Hormone (rBGH) is a controversial drug that forces cows to produce more milk. It is the product of genetic engineering. Monsanto Corporation is the only FDA-approved manufacturer of rBGH.

There are many unresolved human health issues associated with the drug despite FDA approval in 1993. To date, there are no labeling requirements to alert the consumer that (s)he is buying dairy products from cows treated with rBGH. A higher incidence of cattle disease is reported among such animals, resulting in a greater use of antibiotics (which are passed on to the consumer). That's just what our milk supply needs: *more antibiotics!* There are now more than 80 in commercial milk. The animals we eat are fed *thirty* times the number of antibiotics humans use in the U.S.

While the "powers-that-be" in this country have embraced the use of rBGH, European countries have been more cautious: The European Council unanimously adopted a 7-year ban on the product. That ban also prohibits export of rBGH-derived dairy and meat products to the European Union.

There are definitely some dirty dealings surrounding the rBGH issue. A newspaper report stated that "a Canadian government official revealed on national television that Monsanto representatives attempted to bribe Health Canada with $2.5 million in 1990 if it would approve the drug." It was also revealed that a Canadian government official, Leonard Ritter, "formerly in charge of reviewing rBGH approval, concealed from the House of Commons Agriculture Committee his conflict of interest in lobbying for rBGH."

The 10/94 edition of *Dairy Today* indicated that 80% of U.S. consumers have "some level of concern" and 50% are "very concerned" about human health hazards of rBGH-produced products. That concern has grown in recent years, as major networks have given television coverage to this issue in their newscasts. And there appears to be good reason for concern. For more information on the problems associated with rBGH and to join the citizen's campaign against it, contact Food and Water, Inc., 1-800-EAT-SAFE.

TYPES OF CALCIUM

There are many different forms of calcium (and other minerals as well) and it can be mind boggling to walk into a store and note all the different types. My aim in this section is to familiarize you with these different types and to clarify some misleading labeling practices. While I speak of calcium here, what is said will apply to other minerals as well. I am not necessarily advocating the use of calcium supplements by providing this information, but include it for the benefit of those who may choose to use such supplements.

Chelation was previously mentioned. The word is derived from the Greek word "chele," which means "claw." Chelated calcium is therefore bound (or held in a claw-like fashion) to another substance. It is that other substance that is known as the chelating agent, and it determines how efficiently the calcium will be absorbed and utilized. There are two basic forms of calcium — inorganic mineral salts and organic chelates.

Inorganic forms of calcium are found in dolomite, bone meal and oyster shell. These include:

- calcium sulfate
- calcium phosphate
- calcium carbonate

These forms of calcium are called inorganic because the calcium is bound to an inorganic salt: for example, calcium sulphate = calcium (mineral) + sulfate radical (inorganic salt). These inorganic forms of calcium are poorly utilized by the body, with an absorption rate of only about 5-10%. They are, as you might guess, the cheaper forms of calcium. Their use is not recommended.

Organic chelates are much more readily absorbed through the intestinal wall. They include:

- calcium gluconate
- calcium lactate
- calcium citrate
- calcium amino acid chelate
- calcium orotate (no longer readily available)
- calcium ascorbate
- calcium aspartate

These forms of calcium are called organic chelates because the calcium is bound to an organic substance: for example, calcium gluconate = calcium (mineral) + gluconic acid (the organic chelating agent).

In nature, plants chelate inorganic minerals, converting them into organic ones. The human body, given sufficient HCl, can also do some of its own chelating of inorganic minerals. Manufacturers of organic calcium chelates imitate nature in the creation of their supplements. They will start off with an inorganic calcium salt such as calcium phosphate (see # 1, chart 11A). The first step in the process is to separate the calcium from the phosphate molecule (#2). A chelating agent (gluconic acid, for example, referred to as GA, #3) is then added. The gluconic acid, having a natural affinity to the calcium, forms a strong bond with it (#4). The phosphate molecule is then removed from the solution (#5), and we have calcium gluconate, a chelated form of calcium.

Organic chelated calcium is well absorbed by the body. The percentage of absorption will depend upon the chelating agent used, as well as the person's individual biochemistry. Generally speaking, however, the following list gives an approximate idea of absorption rates:

- calcium gluconate   25-30%
- calcium lactate   30-35%
- calcium citrate   30-35%
- calcium amino acid chelate   65-80%
- calcium ascorbate   85%
- calcium aspartate   85%
- calcium methionate   80-90%

Calcium orotate, offering an absorption rate up to 95%, has been removed from the market by FDA dictate. Pure orotic acid causes liver toxicity. The element becomes toxic in the acid environment of the stomach. Enteric coated orotates, however, prevent the release of orotic acid in the stomach and cause no problem.

Now, to reading labels: Can you tell the difference between the calcium content in the two labels below?:

1) Calcium (lactate)   1000 mg.
2) Calcium lactate   1000 mg.

It appears as if both of these contain 1000 mg. of calcium. In fact, only one of them does. That is #1. The word "lactate" in parentheses indicates the source of the calcium. In this case, 1000 mg. represents the actual amount of calcium (from lactate), also known as the amount of "elemental calcium." In example #2, we have 1000 mg. of calcium lactate (no parentheses). This means that *the combined weight* of the

THE CHELATION PROCESS

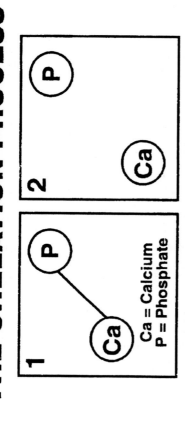

1 Ca = Calcium
P = Phosphate

2

3 GA = Gluconic Acid

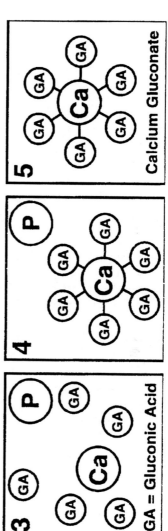

4

5 Calcium Gluconate

Chart 11A

calcium and the lactate is 1000 mg. Since the bulk of this weight is from the lactate, the chelating agent, the amount of elemental calcium present is actually very small, under 100 mg. This kind of labeling can be deceiving. It is tricky but not illegal. If, for any reason, you are seeking a mineral supplement, remember the information given, and look for the amount of the elemental mineral, either stated as such or expressed with the use of parentheses.

In lieu of a store-bought supplement, you may wish to make your own. Try the following: Pour freshly squeezed lemon juice over clean, whole eggs in a wide-mouthed jar. Cover tightly, and refrigerate for no more than 48 hours. Shake gently a few times daily. When bubbling stops, remove the eggs. Their shells will be soft, as their calcium has been leached into the lemon juice, but they can still be used. The lemon mixture you now have is pure calcium citrate. Shake it well, and take no more than one-half teaspoon daily for a period of about 30 days. Note that in this procedure no heat is applied. The calcium therefore is alive and usable by the body.

In view of the preceding information, I hope the next time you hear the word "calcium," you will think in green, leafy terms and not consider the cow. I highly recommend the complete exclusion of all pasteurized and homogenized dairy products from the diet. If you're a cheese-a-holic, consider the substitution of raw, goat's milk cheese and/or soy cheese (both available in health food stores).

THE B VITAMIN COMPLEX

Below are the official members of the family of B vitamins, often called a complex. These do not include the synergistic co-factors that in reality constitute the entire complex:

B1 (thiamine)
B2 (riboflavin)
B3 (niacin)
B6 (pyridoxine)
B12 (cyanocobalamin)
pantothenic acid (B5)
PABA (para-aminobenzoic acid)
choline

inositol
biotin
folic acid

This list also does not include the "step-children" of the B vitamin family listed below, for though elements of the complex, they have not achieved the status of vitamins. For that reason you will not find them present in any commercial multi-vitamin or B complex formulation produced in this country:

B15 (pangamic acid)
B13 (orotic acid)
B17 (laetrile)

Even the two above lists together do not cover the entire complex, for there are additional co-factors.

B13 or orotic acid had been widely and effectively used as a chelating agent prior to discontinuation at FDA mandate. Laetrile (B17), you have no doubt heard, has been used as an alternative treatment for cancer outside of the U.S.

The complex of B vitamins works as a family, synergistically. The elements of the complex occur together in foods, and therefore no one is deficient in any one B vitamin without being deficient to some degree in all of them. Because of their synergistic action, the taking of one or more increases the need for the others not supplied. It is therefore not a good idea to utilize supplements of single B vitamins in the absence of the complex as a whole. Even the complex as formulated, with the 11 vitamins from the first list, is incomplete in the sense that B13, 15 and 17 are missing (as well as the other co-factors, of course). Once again, it begins to look a lot like food might just be our "best medicine," for whole, natural foods are complete and balanced in their nutrient combinations and not subject to FDA regulations in their composition.

Generally speaking, the richest food sources of the B vitamins are liver, yeast, wheat germ and rice polish. The latter two are discarded in the milling process so that the so-called "refined" grains are deficient in B vitamins, even when they are enriched by the addition of a few synthetic vitamins. Once milled, flour loses most of its nutritive value within 18 hours. In the production of flour, all nutrients in the carbohydrate portion of the grain are destroyed. Furthermore, the chlorine dioxide used to bleach the flour is converted by the body to a toxin which has been found to destroy the insulin-producing cells in the pancreas. Is it any wonder that the health of the American people has declined rapidly since the turn of the century with the introduction of pasteurization, homogenization, hydrogenation, chlorination, fluoridation and the milling process?!

B vitamins are meagerly supplied in the SAD, due largely to the refining of grains. The B vitamins are also depleted following a course of antibiotic therapy, for these drugs destroy beneficial intestinal flora that synthesize B vitamins. (These bacteria are best replaced with a rectal implant of lactobacillus bifidus or use of an enteric coated capsule). Also, sleeping pills, insecticides, and estrogen create a condition in the digestive tract that can destroy B vitamins. A high sugar intake will likewise deplete the body of these necessary vitamins. B complex deficiencies are therefore very common in this country today.

The B vitamins play an active role in converting carbohydrates to glucose, which the body needs to produce energy (glucose + oxygen = ATP). As previously mentioned, carbohydrate combustion cannot take place in the absence of B vitamins.

The complex of B vitamins also plays a vital role in the metabolism of fats and protein. These vitamins are essential for the health of the skin, hair, eyes, mouth and liver, as well as for the maintenance of muscle tone in the gastrointestinal tract.

One of the most critical functions of the B complex is its role in the normal functioning of the nervous system. "The presence of B vitamins may be the single most important factor for health of the nerves."[11] Three of the B vitamins — B6, pantothenic acid and niacin — play a particularly important role in reducing stress. Stress is anything that puts an extra load on the body — drugs, chemicals, infections, noise, surgery, fatigue, psychological upset, etc. During the stress response, all nutrients are needed in larger quantities, but the water-soluble vitamins (B complex and C) are particularly subject to depletion, for the body does not store them.

What happens, then, when the B vitamin-depleted body comes under stress? It becomes ill. This has been established in animal studies. It was also demonstrated that animals were able to withstand the stress without falling ill when given a liver supplement, rich in

B vitamins. Since the level of stress in our society is exceedingly high and the intake of B vitamins exceedingly low, we have a losing combination, a natural set-up for disease development.

Although it is rich in B vitamins, the use of liver in the diet is not recommended. The liver filters toxins, and, considering the chemical methods used to promote the growth of animals raised for commercial purposes, you can bet their livers are quite toxic.

B vitamin deficiencies can produce tiredness, irritability, nervousness, depression or even suicidal tendencies, as well as a host of physical symptoms. It is not surprising therefore that vitamin B complex supplementation has been effective in treating a number of ailments. Its use in the field of mental health has been particularly dramatic. Dr. Abram Hoffer of Saskatchewan, Canada was the first to discover that massive doses of B3 (in the form of niacinamide) could help persons suffering from schizophrenia. He gave psychotic patients 1000-3000 mg. at each meal and achieved a recovery rate of 75-85%. Dr. Hoffer has been successfully administering such megavitamin therapy for over 20 years. An entire branch of psychiatry — orthomolecular psychiatry — has developed using this supplemental approach.

One theory as to why large doses of niacin are often effective in treating mental illness is that such patients have a higher than average need for this and other B vitamins not supplied in sufficient quantities in the SAD. For them, deficiencies result in more pronounced symptoms than for the average person.

The orthomolecular approach to psychiatry is certainly an improvement over the traditional drug oriented one. However, megadoses of nutrients, while useful in the short run to correct a deficiency state, are not a viable long-term solution. Large doses of isolated nutrients can have drug-like effects in terms of reducing or eliminating symptoms and, as such, may be useful as an *interim* treatment modality. A cure, however, cannot be claimed until and unless the functioning of the body is brought up to an optimal level, with the normalization of circulation, assimilation, relaxation and elimination, and restoration of the body's ability to regulate itself internally. Getting the body to this point requires considerable dietary refinement and lifestyle change. Vitamin supplementation can be highly stimulatory to the body if used in large doses over a long period of time. Increasingly large doses may be needed to keep us feeling good if the lifestyle changes needed to restore internal regulation have not been achieved. In other words, vitamin supplements would properly play a temporary role in the restoration of health and would most appropriately be a small part of the treatment plan and not the whole of it.

VITAMIN C

Vitamin C helps build connective tissue by maintaining collagen, a protein needed for connective tissue formation in the skin, ligaments and bones. Collagen helps hold together all cells in the body. Because of its role in the facilitation of connective tissue formation in scars, vitamin C is helpful in healing wounds and burns. It also assists in forming red blood cells and preventing hemorrhaging and plays an important role in building immunity, for the white blood cells must be totally saturated with the vitamin to wage an effective war against antigens. Vitamin C increases the body's production and utilization of cortisone, as well as prolonging its effectiveness. Vitamin C, in conjunction with vitamin E and other antioxidants, is required to block spontaneous oxidation reactions, which create chemically reactive free radicals, identified as a causative factor in aging and degenerative disease development.

Vitamin C is found in most fresh fruits and vegetables. Some good natural sources are citrus fruits, guavas, ripe bell peppers and pimentos, the seed pods of wild roses (rose hips), tomato juice, cabbage and fresh strawberries. The RDA (Recommended Daily Allowance) for vitamin C was, for a long time, 60 mg. (100 for smokers), which is a very minimal amount when we consider that an 8 oz. glass of orange juice contains 130 mg. of vitamin C. (The new RDI — Recommended Daily *Intake* — is 75 mg. for women, 90 mg. for men, with an additional 90 mg. for smokers) We must also consider the fact that the vitamin is water-soluble and therefore not stored in the body. Most of it is out of the body in 3-4 hours. It is thus desirable to eat vitamin C-rich foods throughout the day to keep the tissues saturated with this important nutrient.

Vitamin C, like the B vitamins, is needed in extra amounts under stressful conditions. Humans, unlike most animals, do not manufacture their own vitamin C and therefore must obtain it through the diet. Our vitamin C requirements increase dramatically when we're ill.

Adelle Davis tells us that 20-40 times more of the vitamin has to be given during illness to keep the tissues saturated.(12) If we're undergoing drug treatment, it will not be possible to keep the tissues saturated with vitamin C, for every drug on the market destroys the vitamin and continues to do so for up to three weeks after it is taken. Smoking and sugar also destroy vitamin C. All of these things — drugs, smoking, sugar — are stresses on the body. In the stress response, the adrenal glands, which contain large concentrations of vitamin C, are taxed, and the level of adrenal ascorbic acid is rapidly depleted. It is not difficult to see why many of us are deficient in this important vitamin. Many signs that are considered typical of old age — wrinkles, loss of elasticity of the skin, loss of teeth, brittleness of bones — are actually signs of scurvy, a vitamin C deficiency disease. Other signs of deficiency include shortness of breath, bleeding gums, impaired digestion, proneness to dental caries, swollen or painful joints, tendency to bruising, anemia, nosebleeds, lowered resistence to infection and slow healing of wounds and fractures. Breaks in the capillary walls are also signs of vitamin C deficiency. Since clots usually form at the point of the break, vitamin C deficiency can contribute to the onset of heart attacks and strokes.

A group of substances known as the bioflavonoids occur primarily in the pulp of citrus fruits. The bioflavonoids, together with vitamin C, guard the capillaries, prevent bleeding and provide a safe anticoagulant. These biologically active substances are especially concentrated in the white of the rind in citrus. They dilate the capillaries, increasing permeability, allowing absorption of more nutrients from the bloodstream. Vitamin C is 16 times more potent in combination with the bioflavonoids than when taken alone. For this reason, the vitamin C obtained from eating an orange will be more effectively utilized by the body than will the juice of the same orange, especially if the juice was extracted in a conventional citrus juicer. It has been found that there is ten times the concentration of bioflavonoids in the edible portion of the fruit as there is in the strained juice. To include the bioflavonoids in fresh squeezed citrus juice, it is advised that the fruit be peeled, leaving as much of the white rind intact as possible, and then sliced and run through a centrifugal force or hydraulic press type juicer.

The bioflavonoids are also known as vitamin P (think of "P" for pulp). Some of their components are citron, hesperidin, rutin, flavones and flavonals. They are found in fruits and vegetables as companions to vitamin C. *"They are essential for the proper absorption and use of vitamin C."*(13) Think about that statement for a moment: The bioflavonoids are essential for the proper absorption and utilization of vitamin C. With this in mind, how much sense does it make to separate vitamin C from the bioflavonoids with which it naturally occurs? Proponents of the use of synthetic ascorbic acid argue that it is chemically identical to its natural counterpart. While this may be so, it does not contain the essential bioflavonoids, nor the other co-factors of the vitamin C complex. Once again, we are trying to isolate the "active ingredient" and failing to acknowledge the synergistic workings of the natural elements, as well as creating an imbalance of elements in the body. It has already been mentioned that any truly all-natural vitamin C supplement (i.e., one obtained from food sources) would, of necessity, be very low potency, for a 500 mg. tablet of all-natural vitamin C would have to be huge. The higher potency vitamin C tablets may have some food sources in them, but they are primarily composed of synthetic ascorbic acid. While the body's requirements for vitamin C are particularly high at times of stress such as during an illness, and increased consumption of the nutrient is desirable at such times, lower potency natural sources of the vitamin are best used. Concern for the quality of the source should outweigh concern about the quantity of the vitamin ingested. Once again, the amount of the nutrient available to the tissues depends upon the amount utilized or assimilated by the body, which may, and often does, fall short of the amount ingested. Remember: The bioflavonoids, and other co-factors are essential for the proper absorption of vitamin C. During times of illness therefore it is certainly advisable to consume as many vitamin C-rich foods as possible. It would be well therefore to totally exclude concentrated foods, and take in only fresh fruits and vegetables and their juices. The old advice to "get plenty of rest and drink lots of fluid" is certainly good advice; however, be sure those fluids do not consist of pasteurized juices, milk, coffee, tea or tap water. Drink fresh juices. The key word is fresh. Increasing intake of fresh juices during illness will effectively increase the amount of usable vitamin C in the body, assuring saturation of the tissues.

Vitamin C has become a household word, and once again the "more is better" belief has been fostered, backed by supportive re-search. The research supporting vitamin C was funded by Holmes-

LaRoche, the #1 producer of the vitamin. That research, we can be sure, was done with synthetic ascorbic acid. Vitamin C has been considered to be the "active ingredient" in the natural vitamin C complex which includes, but is not limited to, the bioflavonoids.

We've all heard of Dr. Linus Pauling, the man who made vitamin C a household word. Few of us are aware, however, that Dr. Pauling received a $1 million research grant from Holmes-LaRoche to study vitamin C! Few also are aware of the controversy between Dr. Pauling and his former colleague, Dr. Arthur Robinson, regarding experiments on the effects of large doses of vitamin C (in the form of ascorbic acid) on rats. Dr. Robinson, former president of the Linus Pauling Institute of Science in Menlo Park, California, left the Pauling Institute in 1978 after five years of service there. Five years later, in 1983, Dr. Robinson was awarded $575,000 from Dr. Pauling as the net result of a legal battle between the two scientists. The details of this dispute are not widely available. There seems to be a great deal of interest — vested interest — in suppressing them.

A controversial experiment performent by Dr. Robinson is cited by him as the reason he was forced to resign from the Pauling Institute. Dr. Robinson reports that he had done research on mice, which indicated that a "moderate" dose of asorbic acid resulted in an increased incidence of cancer, while a diet of raw fruits and vegetables was very effective against cancer. According to Dr. Robinson:

> The bottom line after three years of research was as follows: When you give mice the equivalent of the 5 or 10 grams a day of vitamin C that Pauling recommends for people, it about doubled the cancer rate. If you give them massive multiple vitamins, it does, too. As you go up in dose range, you near the lethal dose. And just under the lethal dose of vitamin C, there starts to be a suppression of cancer.(14)

Dr. Robinson claims that Dr. Pauling suppressed this data, which indicated that vitamin C was enhancing cancer at the lower doses, only suppressing it at the near lethal dose. He claims that Dr. Pauling destroyed his mice and 19 months later submitted a manuscript to him describing the experiment but not mentioning that the lower vitamin C doses enhanced the cancer, or that the doses that suppressed the cancer were *near lethal*. The paper, he said, submitted to him as a joint venture between himself, Pauling and others, concluded that if the dose were *doubled,* it would provide *complete protection against skin cancer in mice.* Dr. Robinson claimed that the double dose was lethal, and none of the mice had lived. He therefore protested vigorously when this paper was submitted to the Proceedings of the National Academy, and ultimately forced Pauling to withdraw it. Robinson claims, however, that Pauling later published it elsewhere as his own research.(15)

Dr. Robinson is not opposed to the use of vitamin C, but does express a concern regarding the potential damage caused by high doses of the vitamin. Even the "lower" doses referred to by him in his experiment are only low in comparison to the massive ones used, for his range was 5-200 grams (5,000-200,000 mg.). The following statement by Dr. Robinson summarizes and justifies some of his major concerns:

> Large doses of vitamin C have the potential to be very "corrosive" on the body. When large doses of vitamin C react with oxygen in the body, dangerous "breakdown" products are formed. These breakdown products are called peroxides and free radicals.
>
> One of my former colleagues, Dr. Steve Richeimer, and I found that high doses of vitamin C will "oxidize" into free radicals and peroxides and actually destroy protein molecules. When Dr. Richeimer placed large protein molecules in physiological solutions of vitamin C, in a few hours there wasn't any protein left. It was just pieces. The peptide bonds of the protein were broken. Some of the side chains of the amino acids were also destroyed.
>
> In addition, other chemical alterations in the protein occurred.
>
> Later, we found this work was confirmed at an earlier time by Dr. C.W. Orr in 1967. Later confirmation was provided by the work of Dr. F.C. Westall.
>
> Further review of the literature and chemistry showed that the nucleotide base rings of DNA are also destroyed by "vitamin C breakdown products." So now we are not only talking about the potential destruction of body protein, we are also talking about potential genetic damage.
>
> There is still more. Dr. Stich at the University of British Columbia has shown that large doses of vitamin C can have a mutagenic effect on certain types of human cells. Mutagens cause cellular mutations and many of them will cause cancer.(16)

As regards the potential destruction of body protein by vitamin C, Dr. Robinson suggests that this might be the reason the vitamin has antiviral properties — It has the same effect on the protein coats of the viruses.

In addition to the concerns raised by Dr. Robinson, Dr. Alan Goldhamer, D.C., tells us that large doses of vitamin C can trigger a catalytic enzyme known as "vitamin C oxidase," which actually destroys vitamin C in the body. Then, when the large doses of the vitamin are discontinued, scurvy can develop as a result of vitamin C oxidase continuing to destroy the body's vitamin C reserve.[17]   In addition to development of this rebound scurvy, ingestion of megadoses of C can produce diarrhea, raise uric acid levels and decrease urinary pH. This can lead to formation of urinary stones. Also, large doses of vitamin C can interfere with the body's ability to utilize other vitamins, especially B12.

Regarding the optimal daily intake of vitamin C, clearly the experts differ in opinion: anywhere from the 60-80 mg. RDA to the 3,000 -10,000 mg. recommended by Dr. Pauling since the 1960s for healthy people. (He recommended 10,000-20,000 mg. daily for cancer patients). In between those extremes is the 250-500 mg. dosage recommended by Dr. Robinson and other authorities in the nutrition field. This amount can easily be obtained from the diet. It should be borne in mind that vitamin C is well absorbed at low doses, but with higher doses, absorption becomes considerably less efficient.

CHAPTER 12

Beyond Biochemistry: Energy Medicine

*"The secret to coping with stress is simply
to have sufficient energy to meet it."*
Jack Tips

We are entering an age of energy medicine. This age began with the realization that the chemical properties of the body are secondary to energetic ones, not vice versa, as had been previously thought. We are primarily beings of energy whose chemical processes are dependent upon the free flow of that energy through our physical bodies. Findings in the field of physics have confirmed these truths, beginning with Einstein's discovery that matter and energy are basically interchangeable.

Richard Gerber, M.D., elucidated the principles of energy medicine in his 1988 classic *Vibrational Medicine*, wherein he observes that "the vital force creates order in living systems and constantly rebuilds and renews its cellular vehicle of expression."[1] This "vital force" is the basic energy of life — and it can be manipulated for healing purposes through various energetic therapies.

The frequency generator of Royal Rife is an example of energy medicine. So is the color therapy pioneered by Dinshah and Spitler. We have sound therapies (toning, music therapy, etc.) as well. Color and sound, in fact, are related, as every sound has a "matching" color that is vibrationally attuned to it, and vice versa. Homeopathy is another form of vibrational medicine. Here the energetic "signature" of a physical substance is "imprinted" upon a neutral carrier substance, water. Ironically, the greater the dilution, the more potent the medicine. Healing with magnets, gem stones, prayer, laying on of hands and flower, gem stone and other essences may also be considered forms of energy healing, as these directly impact the body's vital force, which, in turn, influences its biochemistry.

To understand the mechanisms and mode of action of these therapies, it is useful to examine the basic underlying principles as expressed in the practice of acupuncture, one of the oldest known forms of subtle energy therapy.

THE TAO

Acupuncture is an ancient Chinese *system* of medicine in which needles are placed in the body at specific points for the purpose of treating illness and/or alleviating pain. It is actually the outgrowth of Taoist philosophy. That philosophy is beautifully articulated in Lao Tsu's sixth century classic, the *Tao Te Ching*. This work is a collection of verses that embodies the philosophy of the Tao. One of my favorites is number seventy-six:

> A man is born gentle and weak.
> At his death he is hard and stiff.
> Green plants are tender and filled with sap.
> At their death they are withered and dry.
>
> Therefore the stiff & unbending is the disciple of death.
> The gentle and yielding is the disciple of life.
>
> Thus an army without flexibility never wins a battle.
> A tree that is unbending is easily broken.
>
> The hard and strong will fall.
> The soft and weak will overcome.

The philosophy of the Tao is well summarized on the back cover of the Feng/English translation of the *Tao Te Ching:*

> The philosophy of Lao Tsu is simple: Accept what is in front of you without wanting the situation to be other than it is. Study the natural order of things, and work with it rather than against it, for to try to change what is only sets up resistance. Nature provides everything without requiring payment or thanks, and also provides for all without discrimination; therefore, let us present the same face to everyone and treat all men as equals, however they may behave. If we watch carefully, we will see that work proceeds more quickly and easily if we stop "trying," if we stop putting in so much extra effort, if we stop looking for results. In the clarity of a still and open mind, truth will be reflected. We will come to appreciate the original meaning of the word "understand," which means "to stand under." We serve whatever or whoever stands before us, without any thought for ourselves. Te — which may be translated as "virtue" or "strength" — lies always in Tao, or "natural law." In other words: Simply be.

In the philosophy of the Tao, the body of man is seen as a sort of small world microcosm which reflects the same laws and the same balance as the universe or macrocosm — "As above, so below."

Major Acupuncture Meridians

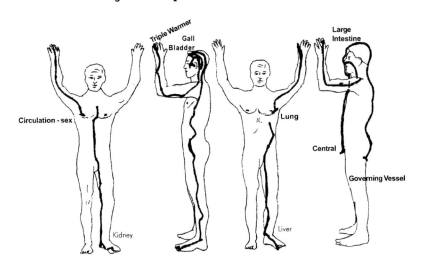

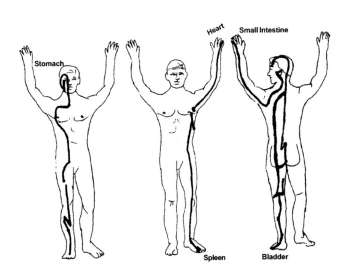

Illustration 12A

CHI, MERIDIANS AND POINTS

The Chinese have a word for that force in the universe that promotes all life. This universal energy they call **chi**. It is chi that animates us, which gives us life and withdraws from the body at the time of death.

Chi does not flow randomly through the body but rather in a patterned sequence through established channels. There are a total of 59 of these energy channels, 12 major ones. They resemble long rivers or streams in the body and are called **meridians**.

Referring to illustration 12A of the twelve major meridians, you will see that many of them are named for organs. The Circulation-Sex meridian is alternately known as the Pericardium meridian. The Triple Warmer (or Three Heater) is related to circulation and to the adrenal and thyroid glands. All but two of these meridians are bilateral — that is, they are duplicated on the opposite side of the body from that which is illustrated. The two unilateral meridians are the "Central" meridian, which runs down the center front of the body from the top of the head to the bottom of the trunk, and the "Governing Vessel," which runs the same course in the back of the body. The Central meridian controls the chi throughout the body. Energy flows through it from bottom to top. Muscle testing will illustrate the power of this meridian, for when the energy is reversed by tracing an imaginary line from the top of the meridian to the bottom with a sweep of the hand, all muscles in the body will weaken. Strength will be regained when the energy flow is restored to its normal bottom-to-top pattern by making a sweep in the opposite direction.

One of the reasons why many Westerners have been skeptical about acupuncture is that these meridians have not appeared to correspond to any known anatomical structures. When I worked in one of the nation's first acupuncture clinics in the 1970s, I read every book on acupuncture I could get my hands on, and most of them asserted that there were no known structures that corresponded to the meridians. Only one made a passing reference to obscure research that verified the existence of meridians as actual physical structures. I didn't again find any reference to this research until I read *Vibrational Medicine* when it came out in 1988. In it, Dr. Gerber described in detail the research conducted in the 1960s by a Korean, Kim Bong Han. This research revealed a fine duct-like tubule system present in the bodies of animals and man which seemed to correspond to the traditional meridian system. Subsequent research verified this correspondence by tracking the movement of radioactive isotopes through the tubule system by high speed CT scan. The isotopes were found to travel the course of traditional acupuncture meridians (as charted 5000 years ago) when injected into an acupuncture point.

When we experience physical or mental stress, the flow of chi or energy is disturbed, and the resulting imbalance can lead to disease. This is a very important concept to grasp: *Energy disturbance can lead to imbalance, which leads to conditions of dis-ease (lack of ease).*

Along the meridians there are close to 1000 points (365 main ones) where the energy channels (meridians) surface near the skin. These are the acupuncture points, which are penetrated with needles in the course of treatment. These points are demonstrably different than other areas of the skin. The electrical resistance is much lower at these points, reflected in a 20-fold drop in reading in galvanic skin response. In the experiment described above, when radioactive isotopes were injected into acupuncture points, the path of the meridians was highlighted, but when the isotopes were injected into other areas of the skin, this did not happen. No discernible pattern emerged.

The meridians are placed where the control of what the Chinese call yin and yang can best be exercised and controlled through needle placement.

YIN/YANG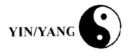

Yin and yang are the two polar forces through which universal energy, chi, manifests itself. They are paired opposites. Yin represents the quiescent, negative female principle. It is symbolized by the dark area of the above symbol. The light area represents the positive, active male principle. Yin is instilled with a multitude of qualities, among which are dark and cold, while yang is light and warm. So yin is female, negative, cold and dark; yang is male, positive, warm and light. While the two forces are opposites, as different poles of the same energy source, they're also complements. One cannot exist without the other. In fact, the essence of one is contained within the other, as is illustrated by the light circle in the dark area and dark one in the light area. So the essence of the female is contained within the male and vice versa. While the Chinese have classified everything in the universe as either yin or yang, it's understood that nothing can be totally yin or yang, only *predominantly* one or the other.

Our state of health is measured by the balance of yin and yang forces in our bodies. Where yang is excessive, the body tends to become overheated; fevers, tension and irritability develop. Yin diseases, on the other hand, are typically accompanied by coldness, depression and weakness.

SHEN AND KO

Some organs of the body are yin. Some are yang. Yang organs are the active, working ones. The yin organs are the passive storage organs. Each organ is influenced by and under the control of one of five elements: fire (heart), earth (spleen), metal (lung), water (kidney) or wood (liver). These elements go through a cycle of creation or generation (shen cycle) in which the five elements stimulate each other as follows:

> **wood creates fire**
> **fire creates earth**
> **earth creates metal**
> **metal creates wood**

The elements also go through a cycle of destruction (ko cycle) in which they inhibit each other:

> **wood destroys earth**
> **earth destroys water**
> **water destroys fire**
> **fire destroys metal**
> **metal destroys wood**

The shen and ko powers are essential to life and must be kept in balance. Disease results when one or more of the five-element functions is either too strong (yin deficient with excess yang) or too weak (yang deficient with excess yin). The diagram below shows the elements, the organs and systems that relate to them, the operation of the shen cycle of creation (large circle with clockwise arrows) and the ko cycle of destruction (which also works clockwise but skips one element, forming a five pointed star).

In these cycles, we can see an implied relationship between the body of man and nature. The concepts of yin and yang hold the notion that man, as all living things, exists in a vast, indivisible whole, which is constantly interacting. To maintain health, mental as well as physical, man must enter into a harmonious relationship with everything else.

Where the life force or chi is polarized and balanced (as it would be through acupuncture treatment), energy flows freely, and the patient's own curative powers are stimulated — so he effectively heals himself. Where chi is balanced and the body is in harmony, the patient will not be a host to germs, blockage, virus or over-emotion. In the Chinese philosophy, even the expression of joy constitutes an imbalance if it is excessive. Excess in any form brings disharmony, blocks chi and causes disease. Excess anger creates too much yang energy, while excess sorrow results in an overabundance of yin.

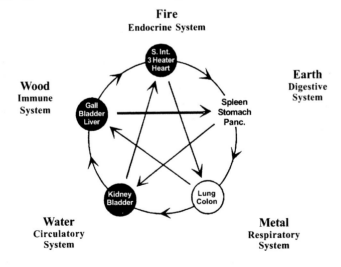

Fire
Endocrine System

Wood
Immune System

Earth
Digestive System

S. Int.
3 Heater
Heart

Gall
Bladder
Liver

Spleen
Stomach
Panc.

Kidney
Bladder

Lung
Colon

Water
Circulatory System

Metal
Respiratory System

SHEN /KO CYCLES

WESTERN SKEPTICISM

There has traditionally been a great deal of skepticism in the West regarding acupuncture. Some claim that successful treatment is the result of the placebo effect — that the patient recovers due to the fact that he *expects* to recover. The fact that something more than the placebo effect is at work is apparent when we consider that acupuncture treatment has been successful both with unconscious patients and with animals, neither of whom has a point-of-view about the outcome! Where unconscious patients are concerned, it's interesting to note also that acupuncture has been used successfully to revive them from a coma.

The skepticism of the Westerner seems to stem largely from his inability to grasp the Chinese explanation of how acupuncture works. It is difficult for the average Westerner to relate to the concept of "chi," for it is not something most of us can see or feel. And, to the Westerner, "Seeing is believing," though many today are awakening to the awareness that the opposite is true: "Believing is seeing," for our beliefs, in a very real sense, shape our reality and bring events into manifestation. Scientists used to think that physical matter generates fields, as evidenced by the electrical activity that can be measured in a person's heart or brain with EKG or EEG. We now know through the findings of modern physics, however, that we once again have it backwards: It is the **fields** that **generate matter.** We are primarily energetic, not physical beings. Our physical properties and processes stem from the activity of the energy that we are, and they are dependent upon this energy. Changes in the activity of energy precede changes in matter and give rise to those changes. Matter and energy, as Einstein taught, are interchangeable. Energy *is* matter vibrating at stepped-up frequency.

CHANGING ATTITUDES

The skepticism about acupuncture that was once widespread in this country seems to be diminishing as Eastern thought permeates our culture. Through such practices as yoga, the martial arts and meditation, Westerners are learning to feel their chi and control it. Most of us are still not able to *see* this energy. However, we hear of people who have this ability.

For centuries, seers, writers, clairvoyants, ancient philosophies and religions have claimed we all possess an invisible energy body (sometimes referred to as an "etheric" body), which can be seen as an aura around the physical body. Today, we have confirmation of the existence of this human double. Scientists have photographed an energy body, an exact counterpart of the material body, only larger, with the outer edges forming a halo or aura around the physical image. Scientific observation of this energy body was made possible through Kirlian photography.

KIRLIAN PHOTOGRAPHY

Kirlian photography, developed in the 1940s in Russia, is a process of capturing an image of a subject's aura by placing them in a high frequency electrical field that illuminates this energy body. It has been verified through Kirlian photography that all living things not only have physical bodies made up of atoms and moleculess but also a counterpart body of energy. Even inanimate objects have an aura, though theirs is emitted as a steady glow, while the aura of a living subject shows movement. Kirlian photography reveals the aura of living bodies to be a swirling mass of colored lights and flares, which changes as the condition (physical, mental, emotional, spiritual) of the subject changes.

Studies of Kirlian photographs of leaves reveal some interesting phenomena: It seems that when a portion of the leaf is cut away, the whole aura remains intact. However, if enough of the leaf (more than 1/3) is cut off, it dies. Energy appears to withdraw from matter at the point of death and disappear. It is a basic law of thermodynamics, however, that "energy is neither created *nor destroyed.*" It does not cease to exist. It simply changes form. The energy that withdraws from matter at death *seems* to disappear, it is believed, due to an increase in vibratory rate, which causes it to enter into another dimension, imperceptible to us. Such speculation is thought-provoking and leads us into esoteric realms.

Getting back to the Kirlian photo of the damaged leaf: The fact that the aura is seen as intact, despite the damage to the physical body of the leaf, may help explain such human experiences as the "phantom limb" phenomenon, where an amputee feels pain or sensation at the site of the severed limb long after healing of the stump has occurred. If our energy body remains whole despite loss of an arm or leg — and our consciousness is connected to that body (as well as to the physical body for as long as we live) — then our sense of the presence of the amputated limb can be understood.

PREDIAGNOSIS

The really exciting thing about Kirlian photography is that it can reveal disease patterns (through changes in the aura) *before* disease conditions manifest in the physical body. This being the case, it is theoretically possible to *prevent* disease by redistributing disturbed energies as seen in Kirlian Photographs. This is exactly what acupuncture does: It redistributes disturbed energies. If energy flow through a meridian is too slow, that meridian is "tonified" through needle placement. The meridian through which energy is flowing too forcefully, on the other hand, is "sedated" through a different placement of needles.

The meridians (or energy channels), you'll recall, are actual physical structures, a system of ducts. They serve the purpose of connecting the physical to the etheric (or energy) body. Dr. Richard Gerber, in *Vibrational Medicine,* refers to them as the "physical/etheric interface." Kim Bong Han, who discovered these ducts, found that their development *preceded* the organization of physical organs in embryonic development. The meridians seem to serve as a sort of spatial guide for organizing the physical form. Kim found in his studies that the meridian system was laid down in baby chicks just 15 *hours* after conception. He demonstrated that the ducts of the meridian system connect with all cell nuclei in the body.

By redistributing disturbed energies in the body before physical symptoms develop, acupuncture can effectively prevent disease, as well as treat actual disease. By balancing energies in the body through acupuncture, dis-ease is prevented and the patient is kept in (or restored to) a state of ease or comfort.

THE DIS-EASE CONCEPT

Our approach to health in this country has traditionally been through disease. We study disease to learn about health. We go to the doctor when we are sick (dis-eased). By that time, energy disturbances have become deeply entrenched. The aura has been out of balance for a long time. To guard against the threat of becoming ill, we purchase "health" insurance, which pays only if we're ill. It would therefore be more aptly called "ill health" insurance!

In many respects, we treat our cars better than our bodies, making sure they have regular overhauls, oil changes, tune-ups and adjustments. We don't seem to realize that our bodies, too, must be aligned, tuned and balanced if they're to function properly.

The Chinese have practiced preventive medicine for the past 5,000 years in the form of Traditional Chinese Medicine (TCM), which includes acupuncture. Their belief that the time to cope with a calamity is *before* it happens is reflected in the proverb, "The superior doctor prevents disease, the mediocre doctor cures imminent disease, and the inferior one cures actual disease." Most doctors in our culture today fail to fit into *any* of these categories! The traditional Chinese emphasis on prevention is further demonstrated by the fact that, in ancient China, the patient paid his doctor as long as he remained well. If he became ill, he was treated without charge! Were we to institute this system in our culture today, the socioeconomic status of our medical doctors would rapidly decline!

PULSE DIAGNOSIS

Chinese preventive medicine is based largely upon pulse diagnosis. To understand this practice, it is important to know that before disease manifests in physical symptoms, there will be for months, or even years beforehand, some physical disturbance that is too slight to cause overt symptoms. Even at this point, the pulse registers definite irregularities, which the doctor of TCM is trained to recognize. The rhythm of the pulse will tell him which part of the body is not functioning or which part is overfunctioning.

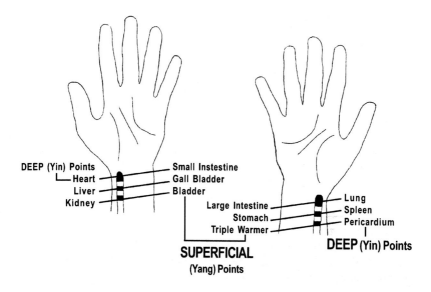

DEEP (Yin) Points
└─ Heart
Liver
Kidney

Small Instestine
Gall Bladder
Bladder

Large Intestine
Stomach
Triple Warmer

SUPERFICIAL
(Yang) Points

Lung
Spleen
Pericardium

DEEP (Yin) Points

The skilled and sensitive doctor of acupuncture can identify past disorders, as well as predict future ones, based upon pulse rhythms. He will feel the wrists of both hands at three points, feeling both deep and shallow pulses on each wrist. Thus he is taking a total of six pulses (three deep, three superficial) on each wrist. The total, twelve, corresponds to the number of major meridians in the body (see illustration above). Irregularities in energy flow through these meridians are reflected in pulse quality. The acupuncture physician is not just feeling the pulse to see if it's fast or slow: S/he's trained to identify over two dozen pulse qualities, among which are "slippery," "floating," "hollow," "knotted" and "scattered." The findings obtained through pulse diagnosis will help determine which meridians are to be sedated and which are to be tonified. Again, the treatment goal in acupuncture is to *redistribute disturbed energies*. And pulse diagnosis is one method of determining the nature of the energy disturbance.

Pulse diagnosis does not yield a *diagnosis* in the sense of giving a name or label to a condition. The acupuncturist is rather concerned with discerning the individual pattern of disharmony in his patient's energy flow. Two patients diagnosed with the same illness by Western standards may nonetheless have dissimilar patterns of disharmony and so would be treated very differently by the doctor of TCM.

A drawback of pulse diagnosis is that it's highly subjective and difficult to learn. In the 1950s, a German medical doctor, Reinhold Voll, developed a device that would measure energy flow through the meridians, displaying that reading in numerical terms on an indicator dial. Readings at the mid-point, 50, indicate balance, while those significantly below 50 reflect the presence of a degenerative condition (and need for tonification of the involved meridian/s). Readings significantly *above* 50 are indicative of an acute condition, reflect the presence of inflammation and a need for sedation of the meridian/s involved. Voll's instrument was known as a Dermatron machine. The design is relatively simple: The patient holds a brass tube connected by a wire to the machine, while the practitioner applies a metal-tipped probe to various points on the subject's fingers and toes (end points of the meridians) to obtain a reading which is displayed numerically.

EAV/EDS ANALYSIS

Over the years, various adaptations of the Voll Dermatron machine have been developed. The basic procedure performed on the machine, often referred to as EAV (Electro-acupuncture According to Voll) or EDS (Electro-Dermal Screening), has been incorporated into computer technology, producing impressive results. These computerized EAV machines, known by various names, such as Computron, Avatar, Interro, Body Scan, are programmed with the frequencies of numerous pathogens and toxins, as well as the frequencies of a number of homeopathic and herbal remedies and various nutritional substances. When these frequencies are placed into the circuit formed between the subject and the machine, the needle will move on the indicator dial, revealing the effect produced in the body by the item whose frequency is being broadcast. In this manner, hidden conditions in the body can be detected, and natural remedies to which the patient would likely respond favorably can be identified. EAV machines are considered experimental devices by the FDA, which has not approved them for clinical use. The name "EAV" is somewhat misleading, for the machine is not at all involved with acupuncture *treatment*, just in measuring chi as it flows through the meridians. This form of analysis, sometimes referred to as ElectroDermal Screening, offers a much more objective assessment of a patient's energetic status than does pulse diagnosis.

THE ORGAN PICTURE

Both EAV analysis and pulse diagnosis give information on energy flow through the meridians. To get the total "organ picture" however, the practitioner of TCM will look for signs on the outside of the body that reveal what's going on inside of it. He'll look for clues in the facial expression, complexion, sound of the voice, sound of the breathing, condition of the tongue. He'll also look at the patient's body build and how he moves and question him about his taste preferences. As the organ picture builds, certain imbalances emerge as prominent.

TWO MEDICAL CULTURES

The sense of connectedness that permeates the philosophy of the Tao underlying acupuncture practice is very much lacking in Western medicine, which takes a much more fragmented approach to healing. This we see represented in the myriad of specialties that abound in Western medicine.

In China today, orthodox Western medicine and TCM (+acupuncture) are taught at the same university. Students of one learn the basics of the other discipline. In some hospitals, doctors of each medical culture work together: The acupuncturist may provide the anesthesia during a surgical procedure and later treat postoperative retention of urine (thus obviating the need for a catheter), while the Western doctor performs the surgery. This kind of cooperation between medical cultures offers the patient the best of both worlds.

Both acupuncture and Western medicine have an impact on the energetics of the body: The former has a direct, intentional impact, while the latter unknowingly affects the body's energies indirectly. *Any* form of treatment will affect the body's energy field and, through it, its chemical processes. Any substance that has healing properties, be it a drug, an herb, a homeopathic remedy, a vitamin or mineral, heals because of the effect of its *fre-quency* (rate of vibration) upon the frequencies of the body. In all instances, **it is the frequency of the mass that heals, not the mass itself.**

Some forms of healing therefore are able to dispense with the mass entirely, having their effect solely through application of pure frequency. This, indeed, would appear to be the highest form of healing, since disease manifests in the energy body long before it expresses in the physical body.

INFLUENCING ENERGY FIELDS

We influence our body's energetic field with every thought we think, every emotion we feel and every action we take. Those actions that influence it most profoundly on a regular basis are connected with the choices we make about what we put into our bodies. Decisions about food have a significant impact on the subtle body. Looking at food from an energetic standpoint, Kirlian photos reveal that the aura of a cooked food item differs radically from that of the same food in its raw state. A head of raw cabbage appears as a lovely blue shape, interlaced with bright flares and beams of white light, while that of a cooked head is a dull, flat blue. The former is alive, the latter dead. The aura around the hands of a person who eats a healthy, well-balanced diet is seen to be intact and clearly defined, while that of a person subsisting largely on junk food will show many breaks and irregularities in configuration.

NOURISHMENT AND BALANCE

The foods that will best nourish our bodies, both the energetic and the physical, are those that are nutrient-dense and grown organically on mineral-rich soils. Such a diet will help provide balance on the physical level. We want to cultivate this same balance in other areas of our life as well — in the mental, emotional and spiritual aspects of our being. Proper fueling of the body, along with detoxification, will allow for clearer mental focus and emotional balance.

The principle of dynamic balance, central to Taoist philosophy and expressed in the practice of acupuncture, is becoming increasingly acknowledged and recognized by Westerners as a critical theme in health maintenance and restoration. It is at the heart of today's holistic health movement, which acknowledges the validity and efficacy of such subtle energy therapies as acupuncture. Such therapies impact the invisible vital force, which dictates the condition of the terrain.

One subtle energy therapy I have found to be of benefit is BodyTalk. Developed in the mid-1990s by Dr. John Veltheim, this synthesis of powerful modalities helps reestablish communication between all parts of the body. It employs gentle touch, tapping and, at times, directed breathing, with the course and sequence of treatments dictated by the body's innate wisdom. Learn more about his system of health care from www.bodytalksystem.com.

NEGATIVITY AND STRESS

Habitual thought patterns affect the energy body profoundly for better or worse. And, that effect is sooner or later made manifest in physical expression. As the late "sleeping prophet," Edgar Cayce, repeatedly told us, "Mind is the builder."

The effect of a negative thought on the body can be dramatically demonstrated through muscle testing. A normally strong muscle will go weak when the subject is asked to think about a past event that s/he found distressing or disturbing. When the mind is focused on a negative thought, negative emotions are triggered. This results not only in reduced muscle strength but also in an imbalance in the energetics and biochemistry of the body, which leads ultimately to disease conditions.

Negativity stresses the body. Such negativity can be triggered by outside events when we allow them to adversely influence our thought processes. Stress does not affect all people equally, for we differ in our ability to "handle" it. There are, however, some generalizations that can be made about the effects of stress upon the human body. Dr. Hans Selye, an expert on the subject of stress and its consequences, has found that even the *slightest strain* on the body (a bruise, an argument, a sudden scare), will cause it to use vitamins and minerals in excess of its normal needs. People who live under constant stress are using excessive amounts of nutritional reserves every day. No matter how ideal their diet, alkaline reserves will be gradually depleted in the face of unrelenting stress.

Stress causes a rise in the body's cortisol levels. The long-term effect of elevated cortisol is a breakdown of the body's muscles, a weakening of bones and harm to the immune system.

While it is advisable for us to minimize the stress in our lives, total elimination of stressors is not generally possible, for these are often the result of circumstances beyond our control. We certainly cannot control the actions of others, but we can influence them through our own behavior and actions, both of which are dictated by our thoughts. And, it is empowering to know that we *choose* our thoughts (though many do so unconsciously). This point is underscored in an unpublished article I wrote many years ago when I first had this awareness. It is reproduced below:

Thinking Makes It So — The Mind-Body Connection

It is a basic tenet of esoteric thought that every encounter is purpose-full and not a matter of chance, that in our reactions to every circumstance do we meet and discover ourselves. As we become alive to this awareness, we come to honor all creatures and events as our teachers. All persons, whether we call them mother, brother, friend, lover or enemy, exist as mirrors that we may view ourselves, for the outer world is the solidified mass created by our habitual thought energy. Form follows thought — and if we dislike some aspect of our life, it can only be permanently changed by adjusting our thinking (the cause), not by manipulating the circumstances (the result).

Look for a moment at the events of your life from a detached perspective, as if you were a spectator. Imagine these events as a movie projected upon a screen. What you are viewing is a direct consequence of your habitual thinking — and, if it is not pleasing to you, you have the option of changing the reel. The "reel" is changed by shifting your perception of reality, changing your thinking, your point-of-view, your perspective, in order to create or project a different image.

You are the *projector* of your reality, which you create with your thoughts. Thoughts are *chosen,* and they give rise to feelings. We automatically choose to react with sorrow to loss in our lives, and it is therapeutic to totally express and discharge that sorrow. But to hold the emotion by fueling it with negative thoughts is weakening to the self, literally draining the body of vital life energy.

It is so very difficult to fully grasp that other people and outside events *do not cause* us to feel what we feel, that there is, indeed, choice involved. When we place the cause outside ourselves, we disown our power and assume a "victim" role. While it may evoke sympathy and commiseration, there is ultimately no satisfaction in it.

The optimist sees the glass as half full. The pessimist sees it as half empty. It is a matter of perspective — and choice. Most of us can look back on life-changing events and see in retrospect they did, indeed, serve a useful purpose and were "for the best," though at the time of their occurrence, we were unable to see beyond our own negative reactions of fear, sorrow, anger, jealousy or whatever. If only our foresight were as clear as our hindsight!

Sit back and watch the movie of your life from a distance. It is then neither a tragedy nor a comedy; it is simply a series of events, void of emotional charge. The ancients say, "Yield and overcome." (Taoist philosophy). There is strength only in flexibility. The tree that stands erect without bending is easily snapped in two by the strong wind. The tree that sways with the wind is not easily broken. Ride the circumstances of your life like the swaying tree with the knowledge that your roots are planted firmly in the calm, strong center of your being.

FEAR AND DESIRE

Of the myriad of feelings to which our thoughts give rise, perhaps the two strongest are fear and desire (an aspect of love). Fear attracts to us that which we do not want, while focused desire, undiluted by fear, will eventually bring forth the desired outcome. While we all desire good health, many of us are kept at a distance from it through fear of illness. Learning to replace this fear with thoughts and images of total wellness can be a vitally important tool for achieving or regaining optimal health. The mind is particularly receptive to such images when it is in a calm, relaxed state, as reflected in balanced brain wave patterns.

Over forty years ago, the late Robert Monroe, author and researcher, developed a powerful tool for influencing states of consciousness and expanding human perception and capabilities through sound. Monroe's patented Hemi-Sync technology consists of complex blends of certain sound frequencies that help the brain move into an optimal state of consciousness for goal attainment. Use of Monroe's Hemi-Sync tapes can serve as a tool to assist the mind in creating conditions of wellness in the body. For more information, contact the Monroe Institute in Virginia, 804-361-1252, or visit their web site at www.monroe-inst.com.

Monroe's Hemi-Sync tapes help to balance right and left hemispheres of the brain so that an equilibrium is established between rational and intuitive thinking processes. Such a balanced mental state helps to dissipate the toxic conditions produced by negative thinking. Physical detoxification can also greatly assist in the process.

THE MINDBODY

In recent years, endocrinologist Deepak Chopra has done much through his teachings to foster an understanding of the relationship between body and mind. He tells us that the body is a physical structure of our thoughts, and emphasizes that if our thinking remains unchanged, so too does the blueprint from which the body is built. Therefore, despite the fact that the various body parts totally renew themselves at frequent intervals (98% new atoms in one year), we tend to hold onto (or re-create) our physical problems.

Dr. Chopra points out that almost all spontaneous cures are preceded by a *dramatic shift in awareness*. When such shift occurs, the patient invariably *knows*, not only that s/he will be healed, but also that the healing force comes from a source within, which also permeates all that is. Less than 1% of all who contract an incurable disease are able to cure themselves in this manner, for they allow their thoughts to be dominated by the "terminally ill" label their doctor has placed on them and therefore are blocked from making the shift in awareness needed to change the outcome. Fear of death becomes stronger than desire to get well. Emotion becomes his/her undoing and makes the terminal prognosis a self-fulfilling prophecy.

For many years, Dr. Robert O. Becker's words from *The Body Electric* have remained in my mind: "Emotions have their effect on the body by modulating the current that directly controls pain and healing." As electrical beings, our emotions express them-selves in the form of actual currents, which influence our per-ception of pain and measurably affect the healing process. Becker found that the key to physical regeneration of severed limbs in salamanders lies in the nature of the electrical activity generated at the site of the wound. The implications of this finding are profound, especially in light of the above statement about emo-tions modulating the current that controls healing.

The power of the mind to influence physiological processes is most dramatically reflected in the phenomenon of "multiple personalities." In this condition, one individual manifests entirely different personalities, as depicted in the classic movie, *The Three Faces of Eve*. Interestingly, there appear to be biochemical changes that accompany the shifts from one personality to another. One personality, for example, may be diabetic, while another is not. Such observations give us much food for thought and ample cause to view healing as a mental, as well as physical, process.

BACK TO THE TERRAIN

Of all the contextual factors that influence the terrain of the human body, the quality of our thinking is perhaps the most important, for as observed, *form follows thought*. Mind is, indeed, the builder, and the "terrain" is more than the cellular environ-ment in the body. It encompasses the energetic blueprint from which the body was created.

Bear in mind, however, that a toxic body tends to generate toxic thoughts, for the physical instrument of the mind, the brain, is negatively impacted by physical toxins. The blood that flows through the body, flows also through the brain. If it does not deliver the needed nutrients and oxygen, the brain cannot begin to grasp or express the knowledge of the indwelling Mind – and the structure that's built will be defective.

Mind is, indeed, the builder, and its creations, our thoughts, have a powerful impact upon the terrain of our bodies.

Afterword

Now, as the new millennium unfolds and ancient truths are brought to light in all disciplines, we come to an awareness of our true nature and our relationship with all of Creation. We come to know that the whole is affected by the changes in its parts, whether that whole be a single body or our collective being, the body of Humanity and All of Life. Nature, our mirror, can sustain and nourish us, or she can destroy us. If the image she reflects to us is a threatening one, we can change that image by dealing with the source of it within our own being, for our collective thought forms create planetary events that we have viewed as "acts of God." May we come to know our God-ness (goodness) and therefore create consciously and constructively so as to restore the Plan and order upon earth!

Our very survival depends upon our willingness and ability to change our perception of reality and thereby change "reality" itself. It's no coincidence that the last millennium saw an increase in both planetary pollution and degenerative disease (pollution of the physical body). The quality of our thinking and integrity of our actions makes a tangible impression upon the terrain of both our bodies and the body of Mother Earth, for better or for worse. We have received our wake-up call. Let us focus on restoration of the terrain in this new millennium, and it will bring new life to our bodies and that of the earth, restoring a sense of connectedness. This connection between the body of man and the body of earth has long been perceived and revered by the natives of our land. Its recognition is reflected in the words attributed to Chief Seattle, when, over 100 years ago, he was faced with the loss of his tribe's land:

We are part of the earth, and it is part of us.
The perfumed flowers are our sisters;
the deer, the horse, the great eagle,
these are our brothers.
The rocky crests, the juices of the meadows,

the body heat of the pony, and man –
all belong to the same family.

So, when the Great Chief in Washington sends word
that he wishes to buy our land, he asks much of us...

If we decide to accept, I will make one condition:
The white man must treat the beasts of this land as his brothers...

Where is man without the beasts?
If the beasts were gone, men would die
from a great loneliness of spirit,
for whatever happens to the beasts
soon happens to man.
All things are connected
like the blood which unites one family.
All things are connected.
Whatever befalls the earth befalls the sons of the earth.

Man did not weave the web of life;
he is merely a strand in it.
Whatever he does to the web,
he does to himself.

NOTES

Chapter 1

(1)   David Perlmutter, "Reclaiming Nature's Message: The Flawed Philosophy of Modern Medicine," *Health & Healing Wisdom Journal*, Volume 23, La Mesa, CA: Price-Pottenger Nutrition Foundation, Fall, 1999, pg.21.
(2)   V.E. Irons, "Detoxify: Enzyme Activity and Rejuvenation," audio taped presentation of National Health Federation convention lecture, 1983.
(3)   Samuel West, D.N., N.D., *The Golden Seven Plus One*, Orem, Utah: Samuel Publishing Company, 1981, pg. 75.
(4)   David G. Williams, *Alternatives*, vol. 7, No. 20, February, 1999, pg. 158.
(5)   Ibid., vol.7, No. 21, March, 1999, pg. 162.
(6)   Dr. Bruce West, "Prescription Drugs: Fourth Leading Cause of Death," *Health Alert*, Vol. 15, No. 7.
(7)   Perlmutter, op.cit., pg. 22.
(8)   Dr. Bruce West, *Health Alert*, Vol. 16, No. 3, March, 1999, pg. 2.
(9)   Walene James, *Immunizations: The Reality Behind the Myth*, New York: Bergin & Garvey,1998, p. 66.
(10)   Dr. Erik Enby, *Hidden Killers*, Hoya, West Germany: Sheehan Communications, 1990, p.16.

Chapter 2

(1)   Dr. David G. Williams, *Alternatives*, Vol. 7, No. 22, April, 1999, pg. 169.
(2)   *Food and Water Journal*, Winter, 2000.
(3)   Tony Webb, et. al. *Food Irradiation: Who Wants It?*, Rochester, Vermont: Thorsons Publishers, Inc., 1987, pg. 68.
(4)   Harvey and Marilyn Diamond, *Fit for Life*, New York: Warner Books, 1987, pg. 126.
(5)   *Food and Water Journal*, Op. cit.

Chapter 3

(1)   David Krough, "Smoking: The Artificial Passion," New York: Freedom & Co., 1991.
(2)   John D. Hamaker and Donald A. Weaver, *The Survival of Civilization*, Burlingame, CA: Hamaker-Weaver Publishers, 1982, pg. 49.

Chapter 5

(1)   Robert S. Mendelsohn, M.D., *Dissent in Medicine. Nine Doctors Speak Out*, Chicago, Illinois: Contemporary Books, Inc., 1985, pg. 148.
(2)   Ibid., pg. 149.
(3)   Ibid., pg. 150
(4)   Anthony Robbins, "Fear Into Power" seminar tape, 1985.
(5)   Ibid.
(6)   Mendelsohn, op. cit., pg. 152.
(7)   Mendelsohn, op.cit., pg. 153.
(8)   Dr. Isadore Rosenfeld, "Don't Worry About Vaccinations," *Parade Magazine*

(Lakeland Ledger), January, 9, 2000, pg.10.

(9)   Richard Leviton, "Who Calls the Shots," *Health Freedom News*, July/Aug., 1989.

(10)   Ibid.

(11)   Mendelsohn, op.cit., pg. 144.

(12)   Mendelsohn, op.cit., pg. 147.

(13)   Hannah Allen, *Don't Get Stuck*, Oldsmar, Florida: Natural Hygiene Press, 1985, pg. 22.

(14)   Leviton, op.cit.

(15)   Robbins, op.cit.

(16)   Tom Finn, Attorney, *Dangers of Compulsory Immunization. How to Legally Avoid Them.* New Port Richey, Florida: Fitness Press, 1983, pg. 13.

(17)   William Randall Kellas, Ph.D. and Andrea Sharon Dworkin, N.D., *Thriving in a Toxic World*, Olivenhain, CA: Professional Preference, 1996, pg. 169.

Chapter 6

(1)   Richard A. Passwater, Ph.D. and Elmer M. Cranton, M.D., *Trace Elements, Hair Analysis and Nutrition.* Keats Publishing, 1983, pg. 258.

(2)   Rev. Hanna Kroeger, MsD., *Old Time Remedies for Modern Ailments,.* Rev.Hanna Kroeger, MsD., 1971, pg. 43.

(3)   Sam Ziff, *Silver Dental Filling: The Toxic Time Bomb*, New York: Aurora Press, 1984, pg. 11.

(4)   Sam Ziff and Michael F. Ziff, D.D.S., *The Hazards of Silver/Mercury Dental Fillings*, Orlando, Florida: BioProbe, Inc., 1985, pg. 15.

(5)   Ibid., pgs. 16, 18.

(6)   Dr. David G. Williams, *Alternatives*, Vol. 3, No. 19, January, 1991.

(7)   *The Main Times*, 4/28/89.

(8)   "Slow Recovery from Palladium Exposure," *Heavy Metal Bulletin*, Vol. 5, Issue 1-2, March, 1999, pg. 32.

(9)   "Are Dental Composites Safe?" *Heavy Metal Bulletin*, Vol. 5-6, Issue 4, 1999-1, 2000, pg. 9.

(10)   "Is There a Renewed Trend Toward Radioactive Compounds in Dental Materials?," *Heavy Metal Bulletin*, Volume 5, Issue 4, 1999-1. 2000, pg. 15.

(11)   Morton Walker, DPM, *Elements of Danger*, Charlottesville, VA: Hampton Roads, 2000,   pg.12.

(12)   Ibd., pg. 214.

Chapter 7

(1)   F. Hollwich and B. Dieckhues, "The Effect of Natural and Artificial Light Via the Eye on the Hormonal and Metabolic Balance of Animal and Man," *Opthalmologica* 180, no. 4 (1980): pp.188-197.

(2)   Darrius Dinshah, *Let There Be Light*, Malaga, New Jersey: Dinshah Health Society, 1985, pg. 9.

Chapter 8

(1)   "The Cellular Telephone Issue," *EcoDwell,* Winter/Spring, 1999, Clearwater, FL: International Institute for Bau-biologie and Ecology, Inc., pg. 1.
(2)   Ibid., pg. 4.
(3)   "The Menace of Electric Smog," *Readers Digest,* January, 1980.
(4)   "Hidden Dangers of Microwave Cooking," *Suncoast/Florida ECO Report,* April/May, 1999, Sarasota, FL.
(5)   Robert O. Becker, M.D. and Gary Selden, *The Body Electric,* New York: Quill, 1985,pg. 324.
(6)   Paul Brodeur, "Annals of Radiation," *New Yorker,* July 9, 1990.

Chapter 9

(1)   Anthony Robbins, "Fear Into Power" and "Nutrition" seminar tapes, 1985.
(2)   Jack Tips, N.D., Ph.D., *The Pro Vita! Plan,* Austin, TX: Apple-A-Day Press, 1993.
(3)   Sally Fallon, *Nourishing Traditions,* San Diego, CA: ProMotion Publishing, 1995.
(4)   Adelle Davis, *Let's Eat Right to Keep Fit,* New York: Harcourt, Brace, Jovanovich, Inc., 1970.
(5)   John Tobe, *Hydrogenation – America's Deadliest Killer,* St. Catherine's, Ontario: Modern Publications, Reg'd 1962.
(6)   Ann Louise Gittleman, *Super Nutrition for Men and the Women Who Love Them,* New York: M. Evans and Co., Inc., 1996.
(7)   Ibid.
(8)   Davis, op. cit., pg. 45.
(9)   *Clinical Pearl News,* August, 1996.
(10)   "Fructose Folly," *Price-Pottenger Nutritional Foundation Health Journal,* vol. 19, No. 1, spring, 1995.
(11)   Fallon, op.cit., pg. 21.
(12)   Nancy Appleton, Ph.D., *Lick the Sugar Habit,* Garden City Park, New York: Avery Publishing Group, 1996.

Chapter 10

(1)   Dr. Richard Murray, D.C., *Applications in Human Nutrition* (clinician's manual), Ste. Genevieve, MO: R. Murray and Associates, Inc.
(2)   Dr. Bruce West, *Health Alert,* Vol. 15, No. 6, pg. 6.
(3)   Ibid.
(4)   Murray, op.cit.
(5)   West, op.cit.
(6)   Dr. Paul Eck, *Healthview Newsletter,* #27-29.
(7)   Kurt Donsbach, Ph.D., D. Sc., N.D., D.C., *Dr. Donsbach Tells You What You Always Wanted to Know About Water,* Huntington Beach, CA: The International Institute of Natural Sciences, 1981, pg. 12.
(8)   "Chlorinated Water Doubles Bladder Cancer Risk," *U.S. News and World Report,* July 29, 1991.
(9)   Vicki L. Elmore, "Speaking About the Dangers of Chlorine," *Healthy and Natural News,* volume 7, Issue 3, pg. 56.
(10)   William Randall Kellas, Ph.D. and Andrea Sharon Dworkin, N.D., *Surviving the Toxic Crisis,* Olivenhain, CA: Professional Preference, 1996, pg. 113.
(11)   Ibid., pg. 110.

(12)   Ibid., pg. 114.
(13)   The John R. Lee, M.D., *Medical Letter*, August, 1999, pg. 1.

Chapter 11

(1)   Guy Abraham, MD, *Health Discoveries Newsletter*, issue #7.
(2)   Louis Kervran, *Biological Transmutations*, Woodstock, New York: Beekman
         Publishers, Inc., 1980.
(3)   Samuel C. West, D.N., N.D., *The Golden Seven Plus One*, Orem, Utah:
         Samuel Publishing Co., 1981.
(4)   Ibid.
(5)   N.W. Walker, D.Sc., *Fresh Vegetable and Fruit Juices*, Phoenix, Arizona:
         O'Sullivan, Woodside and Co., 1936.
(6)   Ibid.
(7)   Bernard Jensen, D.C., *Nature Has a Remedy*, Escondido, CA: Dr. Bernard
         Jensen, 1978.
(8)   Alexander Schauss, M.A., *Diet, Crime and Delinquency*, Berkeley, CA: Parker
         House, 1981.
(9)   Jensen, op.cit.
(10)   *Dairy Goat Journal*, May, 1979.
(11)   John D. Kirschmann, *Nutrition Almanac*, New York: McGraw-Hill Company,
(12)   Adelle Davis, *Let's Eat Right to Keep Fit*, New York: Harcourt, Brace,
         Jovanovich, Inc., 1970.
(13)   Kirschmann, op.cit.
(14)   Dr. John Grauerholz, "The Nobel Fakery of Dr. Linus Pauling," *EIR*, August
         28, 1984.
(15)   Ibid.
(16)   Colin and Loren Chatsworth, "The Great Vitamin C Debate," *The Healthview
         Special Report*, Charlottesville, Virginia: Colin and Loren Chatsworth, 1985.
(17)   Dr. Alan Goldhamer, D.C., "Do You Really Need Vitamin Supplements?,"
         Health Science, November/December, 1989.

Chapter 12

(1)   Richard Gerber, M.D., *Vibrational Medicine*, Santa Fe, New Mexico,
         1988, pg. 41.

BIBLIOGRAPHY

Abrahamson, E.M. and A.W. Pezet. *Body, Mind and Sugar.* New York: Avon Books, 1951.

Aihara, Herman. *Acid and Alkaline.* Oroville, California: George Oshawa Macrobiotic Foundation, 1986.

Airola, Paavo, Ph.D., N.D. *How to Get Well.* Phoenix, Arizona: Health Plus Publishers, 1974.

Allen, Hannah. *Don't Get Stuck.* Oldsmar, Florida: Natural Hygiene Press, 1985.

Appleton, Nancy, Ph.D. *Lick the Sugar Habit.* Garden City Park, NY: Avery Publishing Group, 1996.

Balch, James F. and Phyllis A. *Prescription for Nutritional Healing.* Garden City Park, New York: Avery Publishing Group, 1997.

Banik, Allen E. Dr. *The Choice is Clear.* Raytown, Missouri: Acres U.S.A., 1975.

Batmanghelidj, F., M.D. *Your Body's Many Cries for Water.* Falls Church, VA: Global Health Solutions, 1992.

Becker, Robert O., M.D. and Gary Selden. *The Body Electric.* New York: Quill, 1985.

Bird, Christopher. *The Life and Trials of Gaston Naessens, The Galileo of the Microscope.* St. Lambert, Quebec, Canada: Les Presses de Unniversite de la Personne Inc., 1990.

Black, Dean, Ph.D. *Chinese Healing Principles: Can They Work for Us?* Springville, Utah: Tapestry Press, 1989.

Burroughs, Stanley. *The Master Cleanser.* Auburn, California: Stanley Burroughs, 1976.

Chopra, Deepak, M.D. *Perfect Health: The Complete Mind/Body Program for Identifying and Soothing the Source of Your Body's Reaction.* Harmony Books, 1991.

Clark, Hulda Regehr, Ph.D, N.D. *The Cure for All Diseases.* San Diego, CA: ProMotion Publishing, 1995.

Cousens, Gabriel, M.D. *Spiritual Nutrition and the Rainbow Diet.* Boulder, Colorado: Cassandra Press.

Davis, Adelle. *Let's Eat Right to Keep Fit.* New York: Harcourt, Brace, Jovanovich, Inc., 1970.

Diamond, Harvey and Marilyn. *Fit for Life.* New York: Warner Books, 1987.

Diamond, John, M.D. *Your Body Doesn't Lie.* New York: Warner Books, 1979.

Dinshah, Darrius. *Let There Be Light.* Malaga, New Jersey: Dinshah Health Society, 1985.

Donsbach, Kurt W., Ph.D., D.Sc., N.D., D.C. *D.r Donsbach Tells You What You Always Wanted to Know About Water.* Huntington Beach, California: The International Institute of Natural Health Sciences, 1981.

Duffy, William. *Sugar Blues.* Denver, Colorado: NutriBooks Corporation, 1975.

Enby, Dr. Erik. *Hidden Killers.* Hoya, West-Germany: Sheehan Communications, 1990.

Fallon, Sally. *Nourishing Traditions.* San Diego, CA: ProMotion Publishing, 1995.

Finn, Tom, Attorney. *Dangers of Compulsory Immunizations. How to Legally Avoid Them.* New Port Richey, Florida: Fitness Press, 1983.

Gittleman, Ann Louise, M.S. *Super Nutrition for Men and the Women Who Love Them.* New York: M. Evans and Co., Inc., 1996.

Guyton, Arthur C., M.D. *Textbook of Medical Physiology.* 6th edition, WB. Saunders Co., 1981.

Hamaker, John D. and Donald A. Weaver. *The Survival of Civilization.* Burlingame, CA: Hamaker-Weaver Publications, 1982.

Hensel, Dr. Julius. *Bread From Stones.* Long Creek, South Carolina: Tri-State Press, translated from German 1894.

Honorof, Ida and E. McBean. *Vaccinations The Silent Killer: A Clear and Present Danger.* Sherman Oaks, California: Honor Publications, 1977.

Howell, Dr. Edward. *Enzyme Nutrition. The Food Enzyme Concept.* Wayne, New Jersey: Avery Publishing Group, 1985.

Hume, Ethyl Douglas. *Béchamp or Pasteur? A Lost Chapter in the History of Biology.* London: The C.W. Daniel Company, reprinted 1989 by Health Research, Mokelumne Hill, CA.

James, Walene. *Immunization: The Reality Behind the Myth.* NewYork: Bergin and Garvey, 1988.

Jensen, Bernard. *Nature Has a Remedy.* Escondido, California: Dr. Bernard Jensen, 1978.

Jensen, Dr. Bernard, D.C. *Tissue Cleansing Through Bowel Management.* Escondido, California: Bernard Jensen, 1981.

Kellas, William Randall, Ph.D. and Andrea Sharon Dworkin, N.D. *Surviving The Toxic Crisis.* Olivenhain, CA: Professional Preference, 1996.

Kervran, Louis. *Biological Transmutations.* Woodstock, New York: Beekman Publishers, Inc., 1980.

Kime, Zane R., M.D.. M.S. *Sunlight.* Penryn, California: World Health Publications, 1980.

Kirschmann, John D. with Lavon 1. Dunne. *Nutrition Almanac.* New York: McGraw-Hill Company, Nutrition Search, Inc., 1973.

Kroeger, Hanna, MsD., Rev. *Old lime Remedies for Modern Ailments.* Rev. Hanna Kroeger, MsD., 1971.

Kushi, Michio and Aveline. *Macrobiotic Diet.* Tokyo, New York: Japan Publications, 1985.

Liberman, Jacob, O.D., PhD. *Light, Medicine of the Future.* Santa Fe, New Mexico: Bear and Company, 1991.

Lisa, P.J. *The Great Medical Monopoly Wars.* Huntington Beach, California: International Institute of Natural Health Sciences, Inc., 1986.

Lynes, Barry with John Crane. *The Cancer Cure that Worked.* Toronto, Canada: Marcus Books, 1987.

Manthei, Joseph C., D.C. *Health Through Diet.* Drumore, Pennsylvania: More Excellent Ways Ministries, 1979.

Meinig, George E., D.D.S., F.A.C.D. *Root Canal Cover Up.* Ojai, CA: Bion Publishing, 1993.

Mendelsohn, Robert S., M.D., et al. *Dissent in Medicine. Nine Doctors Speak Out.* Chicago, Illinois: Contemporary Books, Inc., 1985.

Mindell, Earl. *Unsafe at Any Meal.* NewYork: Warner Books, 1987.

Nambudripad, Dr. Devi S., D.C., L.Ac., R.N., Ph.D. *Say Goodbye to Illness.* Buena Park, CA: Delta Publishing Co., 1993.

Oldfield, Harry and Roger Cohill. *The Dark Side of the Brain.* Longmead, Shaftesbury, Dorset, England: Element Books, 1988.

Ott, John N. *Health and Light.* New York: Pocket Books, 1973.

Passwater, Richard A., Ph.D. and Elmer M. Cranton, M.D. *Trace Elements, Hair Analysis and Nutrition.* Keats Publishing, 1983.

Philpott, William H., M.D. and Dwight K. Kalita, Ph.D. *Brain Allergies.* New Canaan, Connecticut: Keats Publishing, Inc.,1980.

Reckeweg, Dr. Hans Heinrich. *Homotoxicology.* Albuquerque, New Mexico: Mexico Publishing Co., Inc. 1984.

Reilly, Harold J., D.Ph.T., D.S. and Ruth Hay Brod. *The Edgar Cayce Handbook for Health Through Drugless Therapy.* New York: McMillan Publishing Company, 1975.

Samuels, Mike, M.D. and Hal Bennett. *The Well Body Book.* New York: Random House/Bookworks, 1973.

Schauss, Alexander, M.A. *Diet, Crime and Delinquency.* Berkeley, California: Parker House,1981.

Schroeder, Henry A., M.D. *The Trace Elements and Man.* Old Greenwich, Connecticut: Devin-Adair Co., 1973.

Stockton, Susan. *Acupuncture: The Manipulation of Subtle Energies, The Restoration of Health.* Winter Haven, FL: Power of One Publishing, 2000.

Stockton, Susan. Beyond Amalgam: *The Hidden Health Hazard Posed by Jawbone Cavitations.* Aurora, CO: Power of One Publishing, 1998.

Tips, Jack, N.D., Ph.D. *The Pro Vita! Plan.* Austin, Texas: Apple-A-Day Press, 1993.

Tobe, John H. *Hydrogenation – America's Deadliest Killer.* St. Catherine's, Ontario: Modem Publications, Reg'd, 1962

Walker, Morton, D.P.M. *Elements of Danger.* Charlottesville, VA: Hampton Roads, 2000.

Walker, N.W., D.Sc. *Fresh Vegetable and Fruit Juices.* Phoenix, Arizona: O'Sullivan, Woodside and Company, 1936.

Webb, Tony, et. al. *Food Irradiation: Who Wants It?* Rochester, Vermont: Thorsons Publishers, Inc., 1987.

Weinberger, Stanley. *Colon Health, Pathway to Health.*

West, Samuel C., D.N., N.D. *The Golden Seven Plus One.* Orem, Utah: Samuel Publishing Company, 1981.

Williams, Dr. Roger, J. *Nutrition Against Disease.* New York: Bantam Books, 1973.

Yiamouyiannis, Dr. John. *Fluoride The Aging Factor.* Delaware, Ohio: Health Action Press, 1986.

Ziff, Sam. *Silver Dental Fillings. The Toxic Time Bomb.* New York: Aurora Press, 1984.

Ziff, Sam and Michael F. Ziff, D.D.S. *The Hazards of Silver/Mercury Dental Fillings.* Orlando, Florida: BioProbe, Inc. 1985.

Facts You Should Know About Water Fluoridation. Mokelumne Hill, California: Health Research.

MAGAZINES AND NEWSLETTERS

Becker, Robert 0., M.D. "Brain Pollution." *Psychology Today*. February, 1979.

Bird, Christopher. "Seaponics and Sonic Bloom—or Sound and Nutrients." *Acres U.S.A.* June, 1985.

Biser, Sam and Loren. "How Increasing Your Energy Affects Your Emotions, Your Personality and Your Sex Life." *The Healthview Newsletter* (#27-29). December, 1981.

Brodeur, Paul. "Annals of Radiation." *New Yorker.* July 9, 1990.

Bruce, Gene. "The Myth of Vegetarian B12." *East/ West Journal.* May, 1988.

Chatsworth, Cohn and Loren. "The Great Vitamin C Debate." *The Healthview Special Report* (newsletter). Charlottesville, Virginia: Colin and Loren Chatsworth. 1985.

Considine, Harvey. "Homogenized Milk, Not Cholesterol Real Villain of Heart Disease." *Dairy Goat Journal.* May, 1979 (from *Acres USA*, 8/78 issue).

Cowley, Geoffrey. "An Electromagnetic Storm." *Newsweek.* July, 10, 1989.

Elmore, Vicki L. "Speaking About the Dangers of Chlorine." *Healthy and Natural News,* vol. 7, Issue 3.

Goldhamer, Alan, D.C. "Do You Really Need Vitamin Supplements? " *Health Science.* November/December, 1989.

Grauerholz, Dr. John. "The Nobel fakery of Linus Pauling." *EIR.* August 28, 1984.

Fels, Harriet. "Fluoridation: Health Measure or Hoax?" *East/West Journal.* October, 1989.

Kotzsch, Ronald. "Bring the Sun Indoors." *East/West Journal.* March, 1989.

Leviton, Richard. "Who Calls the Shots?" *Health Freedom News.* July/August, 1989.

London, Wayne P. "Full Spectrum Classroom Light and Sickness in Pupils." *The Lancet,* volume II. November 21, 1987.

Moore, William H. "Mercurophilia in American Health Care." *Wellness Lifestyle.* May, 1990.

Perlmutter, David, M.D. "Reclaiming Nature's Message: The Flawed Philosophy of Modern Medicine." *Health and Healing Wisdom Journal,* Vol. 23, No. 3. Price-Pottenger Nutrition Foundation, Fall, 1999.

Ponte, Lowell. "The Menace of Electric Smog." *Reader's Digest.* January, 1980.

Rosenfeld, Dr. Isadore. "Don't Worry About Vaccinations." *Parade Magazine* (Lakeland Ledger), Jan. 9, 2000.

Sahelian Ray, M.D. and Donna Gates. "Suddenly Stevia: Rediscovering One Sweet Herb." *Better Nutrition.* February, 2000.

West, Dr. Bruce. *Health Alert.* (Vol. 16, No. 3). March, 1999.

Williams, Dr. David G. *Alternatives.* (Vol. 3, No. 19). January, 1991.

Williams, Dr. David G. *Alternatives* (Vol. 7, No. 20). February, 1999.

Williams, Dr. David G. *Alternatives* (Vol. 7, No. 22). April, 1999.

Wurtman, Richard J. "The Effects of Light on the Human Body." *The Scientific American.* July 1975.

"Blinding Cellphones." *EcoDwell.* Clearwater, FL: International Institute for Bau-biologie & Ecology. Summer/Fall, 1999.

"Everything You Always Wanted to Know About Calcium." Long Beach, California: Nature's Plus, 1986.

"Hidden Dangers of Microwave Cooking." *Suncoast/Florida ECO Report.* Sarasota, Florida, April/May, 1999.

"Slow Recovery from Palladium Exposure." *Heavy Metal Bulletin,* Vol. 5, Issue 1-2, March, 1999.

TAPES
Irons V.E. "Detoxify: Enzyme Activity and Rejuvenation," National Health Federation Convention lecture, 1983.

Pritikin, Nathan. "Lipotoxemia: Nutrition and Degenerative Disease." Santa Monica, California: Pritikin Longevity Center, 1980.

Puharich, Andrija, M.D., LL.D. "The Final Solution to the ELF Problem."

Robbins, Anthony. "Ten Keys to Health" from 'Fear Into Power' and 'Nutrition' seminar, April, 1985.

LECTURE TRANSCRIPT
Morrell, Dr. Franz. "The Bio-Electronic Method of Prof. Vincent" from O.I.C.S. Alumni Association's German ElectroAcupuncture week in July, 1982 at El Rancho Inn, Millbrae, California.

BOOK ORDER FORM

Name (please print) _____

Street Address or P.O. Box _____

City, State, Zip _____

Phone _____

Discount Schedule			Shipping Charges	
2-4 books	-	10%	up to $25.00	- 4.95
5-10 books	-	15%	$25.01 - $50.00	- 6.95
11-15 books	-	20%	$50.01 - $75.00	- 8.95
16-25 books	-	25%	$75.01 - $100	- 10.95
26-35 books	-	30%	$100.01-$150.00	- 12.95
36-50 books	-	35%	$150.01-$200.00	- 15.95
51+ books	-	40%	$200.01+	- 17.95

Retailers: Call for information
regarding trade discounts

*Florida residents please
add 6% sales tax*

For orders outside US call for information.

Qty.	Book Title	Total

Send payment to:

Power of One Publishing
c/o Renew Life
2076 Sunnydale Blvd.
Clearwater, FL 33765-1201
1-800-830-4778, ext. 246

Subtotal	
Tax if Applicable	
Discount	
Shipping	
TOTAL	